Homeopathy in General Practice

'Anecdotal but Significant'

R. A. F. Jack
MB, ChB, FRCGP, FFHom, FBSMDH

Edited by
Janet Gray
MA, MB, BChir, MRCGP, MFHom, DRCOG

BEACONSFIELD PUBLISHERS LTD
Beaconsfield, Bucks, UK

First published 2001

Email: books@beaconsfield-publishers.co.uk
Website: www.beaconsfield-publishers.co.uk

© R. A. F. Jack 2001

British Library Cataloguing in Publication Data
Jack, R. A. F.
   Homeopathy in general practice. – (The Beaconsfield homeopathic library; no. 22)
   1. Homeopathy – Great Britain
   2. Family medicine – Great Britain
   3. Homeopathy – Great Britain – Case studies
   4. Family medicine – Great Britain – Case studies
   I. Title   II. Gray, Janet
   615.5'32'0941

   ISBN 0–906584–51–5

Note: Throughout this book the words 'homeopathic remedy' and 'homeopathic medicine' have the same meaning and are used interchangeably, whereas the word 'drug' refers to conventional medicines. The Latin name of a remedy is printed in italics, while the name of the substance in its crude form is given in ordinary type.

Phototypeset by Gem Graphics, Trenance, Cornwall
in 10 on 12pt Times.
Printed and bound in Great Britain by Halstan & Co. Ltd, Amersham.

Acknowledgements

I have been very hesitant in adding another book on homeopathy to the many excellent ones already in circulation, but have been pressed to do so over some years by several of my colleagues and patients.

I would never have considered embarking on such a project had it not been suggested that suitable help should be obtained. I was doubly fortunate in finding two experienced and sympathetic homeopathic doctors who were prepared to do most of the work for me, and who themselves are talented authors. Dr Marianne Harling began this task by extracting and ordering the relevant material, which I supplied her from my records, including articles that I had published during my working lifetime. The work was then taken further by Dr Janet Gray, who edited the resulting manuscript through many drafts into its present unified form. I feel that I have been very well served in this endeavour, and would like to express to both of them my deep appreciation and gratitude.

I would also like to express my thanks to Dr Mollie Hunton and Mr Nick Churchill for their helpful comments and suggestions on a late draft of the manuscript. My thanks, too, to Mrs Sylvia Mullins, Education Secretary at the Bristol Homeopathic Hospital until April 2000, for her secretarial assistance. Finally I must thank Mr John Churchill, my publisher, who succeeded in persuading me to write the book, and for his patient, persistent encouragement and guidance.

R.A.F.J.

Preface

I was extremely honoured, though somewhat daunted, to be asked to edit a book comprising the lifetime works of Dr Alastair Jack.

As a general practitioner myself, I have always admired Dr Jack's straightforward and down-to-earth approach to the use of homeopathy in his everyday practice. It was a privilege to be able, during the course of compiling and ordering his writings, to get to know his work intimately. I never cease to be amazed how a busy GP could still find the time to meticulously record so many of his cases. As a result of his labour, this book is able to bring to fellow GPs, homeopathic physicians, professional homeopaths and the informed public alike, a practical guide to the use of homeopathy in a myriad of circumstances. It will inspire the confidence to use homeopathic medicines despite the constraints of time.

Dr Jack has a way of using fascinating anecdotes to teach the basic tenets of homeopathic practice, making the study of the subject more easily memorable. He is also refreshingly honest – he often breaks with many of the traditionally accepted rules of homeopathic prescribing, and yet achieves a successful outcome. In this way he challenges us to examine these accepted practices, and not merely to follow slavishly the (often untested) teachings of the past.

I would like to pay tribute to a great homeopathic master.

Dr Janet Gray
MA, MB, BChir, MRCGP, MFHom

Contents

Contents

HOW TO USE THIS BOOK

It is important for the reader to understand that this book is a compilation of the life's work of Dr Jack. Whilst it does not set out to be a teaching manual, it is inevitably a mine of invaluable information on homeopathic methods and technique, and the reader will no doubt pick up useful tips, new remedies and prescribing methods.

A word of warning – Dr Jack has developed his techniques over decades of experience. He is a master of his profession. Often when reading his many case histories the reader may be puzzled at his varied use of potencies and prescribing intervals. He often breaks all the rules – and gets away with it. He often uses high potencies and repeats them more frequently than is generally recommended. Use caution – always prescribe within your range of experience.

There are a few general rules – always stop the remedy on improvement. If no improvement occurs, common sense must be used regarding the length of time the treatment is continued. If the patient is deteriorating, the case must be re-taken or further advice sought. This may, of course, be an aggravation (see below). In a chronic case, if there is no change after a month, again the case must be re-evaluated. If a remedy is continued in the absence of symptoms, the case may be 'proved', that is to say, symptoms of the materia medica of the remedy may develop.

Generally, low potencies (3x to 30c) should be used for 'local' or pathological conditions, and higher potencies (greater than 30c) for conditions in the emotional or 'mind' sphere. High potencies are generally not repeated so often as low potencies, but there are exceptions – you will see that Dr Jack has used *Aconite* 10M for acute fever (pages 6 and 23). This sort of high potency prescribing is safe if the rule for stopping as soon as an amelioration sets in is followed. It must be emphasised that the correct choice of the remedy far outweighs the choice of the potency in cases where the desired potency is not available.

In the case of an aggravation the remedy must be stopped, whereupon the patient should improve spontaneously. If this does not occur after a reasonable interval, the case should be re-taken and a new remedy prescribed.

You will find 'Discussion' sections after certain cases, or groups of cases. I do advise you to pay particular attention to these sections, where you will find 'jewels' of wisdom dropped by the master.

J.G.

Chapter 1

Early Days

I went through my university days at Birmingham without, as far as I can recollect, ever hearing the word homeopathy mentioned. It was only when doing my first house appointment that I was introduced to the subject by someone who subsequently became a very close friend. I treated his approach with the typical suspicion and incredulity that in those days seemed to mark the attitude of most of the members of our profession towards anything unorthodox. 'Why,' I said to myself, 'if homeopathy has done and can do so much, have I never heard of it?' He persuaded me to buy a copy of Boericke's *Materia Medica* with pharmacopoeia, which I kept by and rarely looked at for several years. Each time my thoughts went to it, I begrudged the 55 shillings I spent on it and could ill afford at the time. Now it is my most useful homeopathic book, and I still refer to it regularly.

It was only when doing my first locum, for a doctor who had been urgently admitted to hospital, that I decided to experiment with homeopathy on a patient. I secreted into my bag two boxes of pills, one containing *Aconite*, the other *Belladonna*, and I cautiously tested them on a child with a high temperature. I still remember the curious look on the face of the doctor's wife when I told her that I was going – for the third time that afternoon – to see the same little boy. I remember, too, my excitement and delight at finding how rapidly and effectively the medicine had worked. The mother said, 'My children are always throwing fevers, but I have never seen one settle as quickly as this before, even when using the doctor's medicine' (aspirin). It was a beginning. I then took the Faculty of Homeopathy postgraduate correspondence course and the more I read, the more my interest grew.

At this time I started my own practice in Catshill, in the West Midlands, where I had been living for some years. There was no doctor nearer than two and a half miles away and the village had repeatedly petitioned for a resident doctor. My practice was happily just established before the inception of the National Health Service in 1948. The nearest homeopathic chemist was twelve miles away, in

1

Birmingham, and involved a postal service to obtain their medicines, so I decided to make use of one of the leading chemists in London, as the pills still came by return of post. I got a local carpenter to fit into my visiting case a piece of wood drilled to hold one hundred and twenty one-drachm (3.9 g) tubes (for which he charged me 7s. 6d). I used it for many years and found it a most convenient way of carrying the medicines, with their names written on the cork of each tube. I also acquired a case from the London chemist with two hundred and fifty remedies in granule form, nearly all in the 30c potency. I obtained a set of *Pointers to Common Remedies*, by Dr M.L. Tyler, which I carried in my case and consulted regularly, making many a marginal gloss in them. Later on I bought Kent's *Repertory* and other standard works on homeopathy. (The symptom references, or 'rubrics', throughout this present book are drawn from Kent.)

Thus armed, I got down to studying homeopathy seriously. I would like to point out that in my case it was not so much the metamorphosis from a conventional practice into a homeopathic one, as building up a practice from nothing and discovering that I was practising both therapies equally. Looking back, I consider homeopathy has been a significant factor in the success of my practice. Good homeopathic prescribing is time-consuming, and with a list of nearly three thousand NHS patients scattered over a wide area, I could not have coped using only homeopathy. Often, when pressed for time, I would make a spot diagnosis of the homeopathic remedy, and accompany it with a prescription for a conventional remedy which the patient could get 'in case the pills were not strong enough'. This could save a further visit or night call, but it was gratifying to see how many times the prescription was not presented to a chemist.

I sometimes used homeopathy in conjunction with conventional medicine, for example *Rhus tox.* for arthritis preventing or disturbing sleep, and an analgesic until the *Rhus tox.* worked, as evidenced by freedom from pain on waking in the morning.

I had to alter and adapt my technique, firstly when the NHS started and most of my private patients went, and secondly, as my practice grew and my commitments increased. As to the first, I did notice that in private practice I spent a lot of time with people who only suffered from trivialities, and homeopathy, in certain cases, had the effect of encouraging them to become more introspective and hypochondriacal in their search for strange, rare or peculiar symptoms.

I still smile at my simplicity when I reflect how, on more than one occasion, I spent half an hour case-taking from women whom I thought must be *Pulsatilla* types because of their constantly changing symptoms, and who I have since discovered were histrionic attention-seekers who simply enjoyed being ill, and exaggerated their symptoms, or confabulated. (This, of course, is a symptom picture in itself.)

The second adaptation necessitated by the advent of the National Health Service and the increasing size of my practice was to limit the number of calls, especially night calls. I decided that every family with young children on my list should possess three or four bottles of suitable medicines, labelled as follows:

Aconite 30c. No. 1 fever pills. When hot, thirsty and restless. One every 15 minutes until cool. Also for croup and any emergency.

Belladonna 30c. No. 2 fever pills. When hot but won't drink, and lies still. One every 15 minutes. Also for sore throat or colic.

Ipecacuanha 30c. Cough and cold pills. For simple coughs and colds. One every 4 hours until relief. Stop after three days. Also for nausea or vomiting.

Chamomilla 30c. Pain granules. For frantic pain, earache, teething or colic. Six granules every 15 minutes until relief.

(For the complete list see pages 226–9.)

I would tell the mother that there were five remarkable features about these remedies:

1) They were sugar pills with an infinitesimally small dose of medicine in them, so small that if a pharmacist were to test them he would only find lactose sugar. But, like splitting the atom, the more you divide a thing in a certain way, the more power is released.

   This led to a warning about aggravations – especially with *Ipecacuanha*, where initially the label had no instructions about the maximum number of doses, and several children were made sick by injudiciously continued dosing. It was important to warn the mother to stop the medicine as soon as an improvement had set in.

2) They would not corrupt, nor decay, nor lose their power in half a lifetime.

3) They would work for any age or person and if crushed could be given to an hour-old baby. The tendency was for my patients to regard them as 'kiddies' sweets' and not to try them on adults.

4) They could be administered to a child in its sleep, the child rousing only enough to chew the pill or lick the granule, but remaining semi-conscious.

5) Because they were sweet, children would love them, but even if a child succeeded in getting hold of a bottle and took all its contents, there was no fear of poisoning. (This, incidentally has happened several times. I would tell them of one occasion when a child fed all four bottles into a goldfish tank. But a week later the fish were none the worse and continued to swim about unperturbed.)

In deciding which fever pills to use in a doubtful case, I used the analogy of a bunch of keys. If the first key does not fit the lock, it has harmed neither the key nor the lock, and the next key will probably work. I was impressed by the number of times a mother would bring her child to morning surgery, saying, 'Doctor, this child was like a furnace last night, he was so hot, and we were just going to send for you when we remembered the fever pills. We gave them, and in half an hour he was asleep again. What was he going to get?' To which I might reply, 'Your guess is as good as mine. Whatever he was in for has been prevented from developing, because these pills not only ease, but cure.'

When visiting, I quite often used to administer the patients remedies from their own bottles. One Sunday evening a man asked me to come to his six-month-old screaming baby, as his wife was in tears. In answer to my question he said he was sure they had tried all the different bottles. When I arrived the baby was still screaming and the mother still weeping. The only way she could pacify it was by carrying it round the room. Asked about *Chamomilla* (camomile), it transpired that they had not thought of using it. I gave them some granules from their own bottle, and within half a minute the child was calm – the first time for hours.

The introduction of these home remedies markedly reduced the number of my day calls, whilst night calls became infrequent.

I have been surprised by chance remarks from patients who told me how effective the pills had been in treating conditions where I would not have thought of prescribing them. A young woman came to renew her sister's supply of *Chamomilla* granules and asked if her mother could also have a bottle, as they were the only thing that stopped her headaches. She then confessed that her sister had found them invaluable for her distressing neuralgia, and that she herself found them more effective than aspirin for her own headaches.

To be able to carry two hundred and fifty different medicines in one case was a comfort both to me and my patients. In certain conditions, e.g. coma, convulsions, quinsy or acute gastritis, no allopathic medicine could be administered or retained by mouth, and medication in granule form was ideal.

Early Cases

I once had an urgent call to a child with acute gastroenteritis. The boy was prostrated, and his mother alarmed. He was cold, thirsty for sips of water, and had the typical simultaneous diarrhoea and vomiting. I gave him *Arsenicum album* 30c (white arsenic) and told his mother that by next day, when I called, he would be running about. Two hours after I left, he asked for, ate and kept down, part of his father's cooked dinner. He had no more diarrhoea or sickness. His mother was amazed.

Only three times can I remember admitting a child to hospital with measles, out of three hundred and twenty-five cases notified in my first ten years of practice. In each case they were under one year old. *Pulsatilla* and *Sulphur* were usually most effective. Later I discovered the benefit of using *Euphrasia* in the prodromal stage of the infection. Indeed, it became a rare event to admit a child of any age to hospital except for an acute abdomen, and this I attribute to the fact that they were given *Aconite* or *Belladonna* at the onset of their febrile illness.

I recollect being on call for a colleague who warned me of a publican's wife who would almost certainly send for me. She had suffered from headaches intermittently for months, and on this occasion had been in bed for several days with one. She was, he said, a typical neurotic; she had done the rounds of the specialists and neither they, nor he, could do anything for her. Sure enough, a most pressing call came in the afternoon. On arrival I found an agitated husband who almost defiantly told me to go upstairs quietly, as his wife was going 'crazy' with her headache. I found the woman lying immobile in bed with her hands pressed firmly to her forehead. The curtains were drawn.

The headache was thumping, relieved by strong pressure, and worse for noise, light, touch, even the vibrations of my footsteps on the stairs and in her room. She would not reply to me, her husband had to supply the answers to my questions. I gave her one pill of *Bryonia* 12c to suck. She would not open the eyes or move her hands to receive it. I had to put it in her mouth. In less than half a minute she spoke for the first time and called her husband, saying, 'It's all going. What wonderful relief!' I left her with two more pills in case of relapse, and her husband was much more friendly and polite as we went downstairs. Next morning a very grateful doctor phoned to thank me and asked about the remedy, and where he could obtain a further supply. That was his first introduction to homeopathy.

During the Asian flu epidemic of 1957, I visited over four hundred cases. A Ministry of Health circular warned us what to expect. It was a classical description of a *Belladonna* proving. My only addition to this excellent remedy picture would have been to include photophobia and conjunctival injection. Of the patients I visited, one half had already been taking the fever pills as indicated, with considerable relief. I found that *Belladonna* not only rapidly reduced the temperature but also controlled the abdominal spasms and afternoon pyrexia which often persisted for a week or more as sequelae. I was able to verify that high potencies were far more effective than low, and when my supply of a remedy was running out I got the patients to dissolve two pills in a glass of water and take dessertspoonful doses, which worked very well. Four of my own children went down with the flu, in each case their temperature exceeded 40°C (104°F). *Belladonna* 200c quickly brought them out of their delirium and cooled them down. We did not have a single night up with any of them.

In the circular referred to above it was stated that 'the temperature would rise rapidly to 103–104°F (39.5–40°C) and remain up for 48–72 hours'. In no case that I treated did the temperature remain as high as that for more than a few hours after administration of the homeopathic remedy.

I will quote two examples. In the early weeks of the epidemic, on my half-day, I received two similar calls from the same outlying district. In each case the husband phoned for his wife, who was very feverish and restless. In both cases they thought they had fever pills somewhere in the house, and agreed to go on giving them until I called. When I arrived late that evening at the first house I found the woman had had a good sweat and was cool. She had only taken fever pills. At the second house, the woman lay in bed, restless and panting for breath, with a temperature of 106°F (41°C) – the highest I recall having seen except in terminal conditions. The husband said that he had found the fever pill bottles were empty, and he was about to send for me. To complicate matters, his wife could not tolerate aspirin in any form. In this case I gave *Aconite* 10M every half hour in view of her restlessness. I left at 10p.m. and saw her next day at noon. She had a restless night, but her temperature was down to 100°F (37.8°C). She was feeling much better now, and wanted to sleep. Next day she was apyrexial. I wonder what conventional medicine could have offered in this case apart from tepid sponging.

As I have already mentioned, I often found it advantageous and even necessary to use conventional medicine, as do many other doctors practising homeopathy under the National Health Service. One reason was that successful prescribing in homeopathy is time-consuming, and in a crowded surgery it is impracticable to give the necessary time to every patient to decide which homeopathic remedy they require. Nevertheless, there are many occasions when it is possible to find a homeopathic remedy which will be far more effective than its conventional counterpart, or where no effective conventional remedy exists. This book consists of numerous such case histories which I recorded, either on tape or in writing, throughout more than fifty years in medical practice.

Chapter 2

Getting Started

HOMEOPATHIC MEDICINES

Homeopathic medicines are prepared as tinctures, tablets, granules or powders. They contain a small amount of medicine which has been treated by repeated dilution, with vigorous shaking (succussion) at each stage of the dilution. This process is called 'potentisation'. The substances used are prepared from plant, animal and chemical products, and are described by their Latin names to facilitate international use. They can be used in conjunction with ordinary conventional medicines, although their action may be less effective in such a case; this is understandable, as the homeopathic medicine is thought to act on the body's autoregulatory mechanisms, and if these are already being influenced by powerful drugs the action of the homeopathic medicine may be vitiated. For years I followed the accepted teaching of those days, that one only prescribed one form of treatment at a time. After a lifetime's use of homeopathy in general practice I have discovered, along with many of my experienced colleagues, that homeopathic treatment can be a very effective additional form of therapy, as will be evident in several of the cases recorded in subsequent chapters.

This is a fundamental issue, with important implications, especially when treating patients with chronic illnesses who have been having conventional medication for years.

There was a time when certain homeopaths insisted categorically that their patients must stop taking all conventional medicines before starting homeopathic treatment. This could have had disastrous effects, for example in the case of maintenance therapy for deficiency diseases (insulin, thyroxine, etc.), or steroids or other life-support drugs. To authorise or condone such advice was reprehensible, and nowadays could be construed as malpraxis. A homeopathic consultant does not usually have the primary care of the patient, and the general practitioner at the other end would be left to deal with any subsequent emergency that had been precipitated by such irresponsible advice.

Happily this situation need not arise. In my letter to GPs I routinely inform them that I have instructed their patient to continue taking whatever conventional medicine is being prescribed, as homeopathic treatment will only be an additional form of therapy. I suggest that if the homeopathic medicine is seen to be working, the GP may find that the dose of the conventional medicine can safely be reduced, but that would be his or her decision. In practice this has frequently happened, involving the reduction of the dose of analgesics, antihistamines, antibiotics, and even steroids.

Admittedly, patients have independently decided to reduce, or even discontinue, their conventional medication without my knowledge or consent, and have got away with it, but it was inadvisable (see the case of hypertension treated with *Lycopodium* and *Spartium*, pages 103–10).

On several occasions whilst I was a GP, I successfully treated my own NHS patients who suffered from heart failure by substituting digoxin and diuretics with *Crataegus*. They were very pleased with their own symptomatic improvement, which was sustained, but I was able to monitor them closely and was always available for advice if their condition deteriorated.

Homeopathic Medicines have Certain Unique Qualities

Acceptability

These medicated tablets are universally popular. The most nervous or resistant child will take them after tasting one. The children in my district called them 'sweeties' and enjoyed visiting surgery in the hope of being given one. They are ideal for the occasional child who resolutely refuses every other form of medication, or for adults who decline to take 'drugs'.

Shelf-Life

Homeopathic medicines, if properly prepared and stored in the dark in screw-capped glass bottles, keep their strength for years. However, they must not be contaminated by coming into contact with volatile oils, camphor, embrocations or similar substances, which inactivate them. Homeopathic tablets of one medicine must not be put into a bottle that has previously contained a different homeopathic medicine. The manufacturing chemists who supply these medicines usually give detailed instructions about how they should be kept and administered. The pharmacist's initial outlay in stocking them is minimal, as is the shelf room required to store them.

Administration

Homeopathic medicines can often be given orally when a conventional equivalent would have to be given parenterally; for example, in cases of repeated vomiting, quinsy, syncope, coma and epilepsy, or during sleep. A few medicated granules can be placed, dry, on the tongue or inside the lips. The medicine is rapidly absorbed through the buccal mucosa.

Speed of Action

In many acute conditions or emergencies the rapidity of action of homeopathic medicines is astonishing. *Aconite* and *Belladonna* act as a febrifuge far more quickly than paracetamol, and will, when indicated, start to bring down the temperature in a few minutes. In migraine and hay fever the speed of action can be equally dramatic. A screaming babe which has been crying for hours will become quiet, and even start smiling and gurgling, within minutes of receiving potentised *Chamomilla* – when *Chamomilla* is the indicated remedy.

Economy

The average homeopathic prescription costs the NHS less than half the price of a conventional equivalent. All homeopathic medicines can be prescribed on the NHS.

Effectiveness

Gratifying cures have been effected by homeopathic medicines when conventional medicines seemed to have nothing further to offer. This book records many case histories of patients with varying conditions. Homeopathic treatment can abort shingles, greatly improve intractable migraine, lifelong eczema, facial acne, hayfever and resistant allergies, asthma, menopausal flushes and sweats, impotence and even photosensitivity. It is the ideal treatment for the many patients with less serious or disabling conditions, who fill a doctor's surgery and for whom conventional treatment can often only palliate – people suffering from catarrh, including eustachian catarrh, feverish colds or flu, recurrent colds, pharyngitis, buccal ulcers, cervical lymphadenopathy, recurrent boils or skin sepsis, dyspepsia, and so on.

In chronic diseases, where spontaneous remissions are rare or unlikely, homeopathic medicine can still palliate and improve the quality of life, either when given alone or in addition to conventional medicines. In fact, there are few medical conditions for which homeopathy cannot offer some help. Of course, there is still a need for conventional medicine; for hospitals, with their specialist expertise and investigatory procedures; for replacement therapy in deficiency diseases; for surgery. Homeopathy complements conventional medicine. On many occasions, however, patients have been taken off the operating list, when awaiting surgery, following successful treatment with homeopathic medicines. Usually these have only been cases for minor surgery, such as haemorrhoids, varicose veins, antrum washouts, and so on, but some have even escaped major surgery for conditions such as peptic ulcers or ulcerative colitis.

Toxicity

Homeopathic medicines are non-toxic and are not known to produce iatrogenic side effects. (Nor have there been any recorded cases of teratogenic or embryotoxic abnormality induced by homeopathic medicines.) This is relevant in the light of a recent survey which showed that one in ten of all admissions to geriatric departments in the UK were caused wholly or partly by drug side effects.

Every conventional drug is potentially dangerous, and you must ask yourself, 'What could go wrong if I use it, and in the event of an untoward reaction, what could I then do?' This does not in general apply to homeopathic medicines, although they can produce a serious aggravation when used in high potency, especially in skin conditions.

Constant and Unvarying

Homeopathy has not altered in the last two hundred years since it was first taught by Hahnemann; the pharmacology of its medicines has not altered. In contrast, we are told that the half-life of a modern drug is ten years! Compare the changes in the treatment of hypertension in the last twenty years. At one time I was receiving information on twenty or so new drug preparations monthly, many of which were destined to be withdrawn, or replaced, within a few years. As one GP used to say to the drug company representative who was introducing a new product: 'If it is still in use in a year's time, I will try it.'

Stimulating

Homeopathy is a most absorbing, interesting and rewarding study. You are searching for a substance whose materia medica represents the symptomatology of the patient. It is true that this involves learning afresh, and in greater detail, the toxicology of many medicines, but this need only be done gradually. Although experienced homeopaths are familiar with several hundred homeopathic medicines, and regularly use over a hundred different ones, much can be done with a working knowledge of only a score or more. If you spend five minutes reading up one of the commoner medicines, the chances are (in general practice) that within a day or two you will meet a patient whose symptoms are crying out for that very remedy. Then you prescribe it with confidence, are gratified to see it work, and are encouraged to experiment further.

If you are unsure as to whether a remedy is the indicated one, a safe expedient is to give a few doses of the homeopathic medicine and a prescription for a conventional alternative, with instructions to use the homeopathic tablets first, and – only if they 'are not strong enough' – to have the prescription dispensed. If the homeopathic medicine does work it is less likely to be due to suggestion, since doubt as to its efficacy will have been raised in the patient's mind.

HOME REMEDIES

For the busy GP, a convenient way of introducing homeopathy into his or her practice is to utilise a set of home remedies (see 'Home Remedy Kit', pages 226–9), comprising a basic set of about two dozen of the most commonly used remedies for acute conditions. These labelled bottles give not only the name of the remedy, but also the homeopathic indications for using it. This latter is important, because homeopathic prescribing has to be 'tailor made', relating to the whole patient rather than just to the disease. Thus four consecutive cases of flu might require four different medicines, depending on how each patient has reacted to the influenza virus infection. Happily, with flu it usually happens that in any one epidemic most patients display the same symptoms, so that most will in fact benefit from one homeopathic medicine.

The next step is to let the patients have their own small supply of medicines for first-aid or home use. Start with your own family: many a doctor has told me that it was his wife who was the first to test the medicines, and her initial success and enthusiasm prompted him to start using them in his practice. Then move on to the most demanding families, or those at a distance, or those that have the most illness. I issued these sets of medicines regularly to my NHS patients. Routinely, every family that joined the practice was invited to have their own supply of homeopathic medicines, together with an instruction sheet.

Getting Started

HOMEOPATHIC PRESCRIBING

Homeopathic treatment involves taking a history of the case and a detailed examination of the patient, in the conventional way; but it differs from conventional treatment inasmuch as it uses the principle of treating the whole patient rather than that person's individual symptoms.

An analogy from one of the few forms of conventional prescribing where this principle is applied will illustrate the point. Consider a case of depressive illness. It is well recognised that this may present with various intractable somatic symptoms such as lassitude, dyspnoea, gastralgia, constipation, amenorrhoea, insomnia, or even severe headache or muscular pains. The usual palliative treatments, including tranquillisers, fail to help, and it may be months before the diagnosis of depression is made. Using current conventional therapy, little or no relief will be obtained until the required antidepressive agent is prescribed. The patient is predominantly concerned about his one particular somatic symptom: you treat his general and mental condition, anticipating a predictable improvement in the next few weeks. Similarly, the pleomorphic symptoms of diabetes will only be controlled by treating the underlying disorder.

Homeopathic nomenclature also uses three words – 'Mentals', 'Generals' and 'Particulars' – in describing symptoms, and attaches importance to them in that order.

Mentals

This refers to the mental make-up of the patient, with variations of affect, disposition and attitude. It is well recognised that certain illnesses (e.g. jaundice, with its 'melancholia') and certain drugs (e.g. gold injections) make the patient depressed. Homeopathic provings have shown that many drugs affect the mental state of a patient, as in the cases in Chapter 4.

Hahnemann quoted many examples of effective therapies used by the medical authorities of his day that were based on the homeopathic principle, including the use of hyoscyamus (henbane) in treating mania – before the advent of phenothiazines it was the treatment of choice in our mental hospitals. Yet an overdose of henbane makes a person suspicious, fearful, jealous and paranoid. Larger doses produce confusion, acute mania and even acute delirium.

The crude substance may affect sleep (even dreams), memory, balance, sight. They disturb the appetite, causing unusual cravings or

13

aversions; e.g. silver nitrate makes a person impulsive and intolerant of heat, and produces flatulent dyspepsia with an irresistible craving for sweet things.

Generals

Substances also affect the patient's general condition, so that he may become intolerant of the cold (arsenic) or the heat (bee sting) or damp (sodium sulphate) or of a north-east wind (calcium sulphide). Or they may cause a feeling of great weakness (potassium carbonate and other potassium salts, as in hypokalaemia).

Particulars

These symptoms generally refer to the action of some drugs on different parts of the body. For example, bryony selects the serous membranes and pleura, producing synovitis and pleurodynia; phosphorus affects the stomach, giving rise to an intense craving for cold drinks which are promptly vomited back again; copper causes cramps, and lead poisoning results in colic and wrist-drop.

'Modalities' is another term employed in homeopathy and is used to qualify symptoms, e.g. 'worse for movement' (written '< movement') or 'better for pressure' ('> pressure') or 'better for applied heat', etc.

I have derived great benefit from the list of 'remedies aggravated by heat and aggravated by cold' in Dr Gibson Miller's *Relationship of Remedies*. 'It is worth while having the list of 'hot' medicines at one's fingertips, and then by elimination one recognises the neutral and the cold ones. Kent, in the 'Generals' section of his *Repertory*, includes more medicines than those chosen by Dr Gibson Miller who, (presumably for practical purposes) limited his list to twelve 'hot' remedies in capitals, and twenty-four in italics. I mentally list them opposite – in a way probably 'strangely peculiar' to my way of memorising data.

Looking at this 'hot' list, you will notice that, as a memory aid:

1) I have paired the first twelve remedies in capitals, because in five out of six cases the pairs begin with the same letter.
2) *Platina* and *Sabina* nearly rhyme; this stops you inadvertently confusing *Sabina* with, say, *Sabadilla*.
3) In the second (italic) list I have put *Hamamelis* and *Opium* out of alphabetical order to make the mnemonic H-O-G!

14

Remedies Aggravated by Heat ('Hot Remedies')

APIS	*Aesculus hipp.*
ARGENTUM NIT.	*Allium cepa*
	Aloe soc.
FLUORIC ACID	*Asafoetida*
IODUM	*Aurum mur.*
	Aurum iod.
KALI IOD.	
KALI SULPH.	*Bryonia*
	Caladium
NATRUM MUR.	*Calc. iod.*
NATRUM SULPH.	*Calc. sulph.*
	Coccus cacti
PLATINA	*Crocus*
PULSATILLA	
	Drosera
SABINA	
SECALE	*Hamamelis*
	Opium
	Gratiola
	Lachesis
	Ledum
	Lilium tig.
	Lycopodium
	Spongia
	Sulphur
	Sulphur iod.

Vespa

The entire list begins with a bee (*Apis*) and ends with a wasp (*Vespa*), and the list in capitals terminates with *Secale* (ergot), which makes you feel as though both bees and wasps (and ants) were crawling over your skin (formication).

Dr Gibson Miller, who extracted this list from Kent's works, also classifies all the important remedies predominantly aggravated by cold. He lists twenty-nine in capitals and sixty-five in italics – which explains why I prefer to learn the 'hot' list instead of the 'cold'! There are also another sixteen 'also-rans' in plain type, but when the general symptom is as inconspicuous as to be only in plain type, I don't find it of much practical value.

These aggravations apply to general and not to particular symptoms (the general symptom being one introduced by 'I' and the particular by 'my'). Thus, 'My toothache is worse after a warm drink, but I feel better in a warm room, and worse in the cold', places *Chamomilla* in the group of cold remedies. *Mercury* and a few other remedies are aggravated by heat in acute conditions and by cold in chronic conditions. Many medicines in common use do not figure on either list, because they do not have a pronounced hot or cold modality.

The first and most obvious use of this list is that where one finds a strong general symptom of aggravation from either heat or cold, one can usually safely eliminate all the remedies in the opposite list. For example, if you were treating a patient with migraine, and the indicated remedy boiled down to either *Natrum mur.* or *Silica*, you would find that *Natrum mur.* is in the 'hot' list in bold type, whereas *Silica* is in equally bold type in the 'cold' list. This makes the choice easier in assessing the totality of the symptoms.

Notice that *Secale* is in capitals in the 'hot list' – one of our best remedies for hypothermia in elderly, scrawny women. Objectively they feel like a block of ice, and you can diagnose the condition without a low-reading thermometer, simply by placing your hand in the axilla; it is immediately apparent how cold they are. Subjectively they feel hot, and cannot tolerate any external heat – indeed a strange symptom.

I had an aged aunt who some years ago was found to be in hypothermia. It was during a freeze-up in winter, yet she had all the windows of her house open and didn't want any heating on. As she lived alone we had to hijack her to our house, and despite the fact that it was snowing and the temperature was sub-zero, she insisted on having the car heater off and the car windows open.

Later, after she had recovered, she developed faecal incontinence (of which she was oblivious) and as she was still aggravated by external heat, was given *Aloe* – also in the 'hot' list – in the 30th potency, which rapidly cured her condition.

Surprisingly, further scanning of the list reveals the interesting fact that Dr Gibson Miller only put the *Sulphur* patient in the second column, whereas he put the *Natrum mur.* and *Pulsatilla* patients (who both feel 'chilly') in the first.

Iodum and *iodides* account for four of the thirty-six remedies aggravated by heat; there are no iodides in the 'cold' list.

The addition of a sulphate to a 'cold' remedy converts it to a 'hot' remedy on three occasions – *Kali sulph.*, *Nat. sulph.* and *Calc. sulph.*

The two exceptions to this rule are *Aurum sulph.* and *Carboneum sulph.*, which are predominantly 'cold'.

Fluoric acid and *Picric acid* are the only acid remedies aggravated by heat.

In the 'Modalities' section of the Repertory the aggravations are listed before the ameliorations.

DIFFERENCES BETWEEN HOMEOPATHIC AND CONVENTIONAL PRESCRIBING

The homeopathic doctor has to assess the whole patient, with his mental, general and particular symptoms, and find a corresponding remedy picture. Obviously, if he can isolate a unique or peculiarly outstanding symptom that few drugs in toxic doses can produce, his task is simplified.

In a police search, if the description states 'right thumb missing' or 'tattoo on left arm', the hunt for the suspect is made much easier. In the same way, if we find a prominent, unusual symptom, the list of possible remedies is immediately shortened, as only a few drugs will produce that symptom in their provings.

Suppose that the patient simply complains of nausea. It would be profitless to hunt in the repertory among the hundreds of medicines that cause this. Most drugs in toxic doses ultimately do cause nausea. If, however, questioning reveals that the patient has a headache, has become extremely irritable and unsociable, is offended at the most harmless word (like a 'bear with a sore head') and is hypersensitive to noise and smells; if he feels unusually chilly, has a sore throat, has piles, an unsatisfactory bowel function ('false alarms', ineffectual urging), cannot sleep at night and is worse in the mornings, then *Nux vomica* is probably indicated. Here the choice is made by his mental and general symptoms rather than by the particular one of nausea.

Homeopathic prescribing differs from conventional prescribing in that only one medicine is given.

Conventional treatment nowadays tends more to polypharmacy, so that the patient mentioned above might leave the surgery with prescriptions for several drugs, for example:

1) an analgesic for his headache,
2) lozenges for his sore throat,
3) an antacid for his dyspepsia,
4) a laxative for his constipation,
5) an ointment for his piles,

6) a tranquilliser for his irritability, and
7) a hypnotic for his insomnia.

How much simpler to give one medicine that covers the totality of his symptoms, i.e. *Nux vomica*.

It must be freely admitted that it is by no means always possible to find one single medicine which corresponds in this way; and we have our failures when prescribing homeopathic medicines, as we do when using conventional therapy. But there is no risk of drug interaction, nor, as already mentioned, have any iatrogenic, teratogenic or embryotoxic effects been reported.

Homeopathic medicines do not suppress symptoms – the dose is too small; they can only work by stimulating the body. How often do we explain to our patients that time will heal, or that the child will outgrow the catarrhal stage, or that no antibiotic is effective against viral infections? We withhold antibiotics, give palliative treatment, and let the body develop and mobilise its own defences. It is at this level that homeopathic medicine is thought to work.

In treating chronic skin lesions, the use of strong topical applications, particularly steroids, only suppresses the condition, which frequently flares up again when the treatment is discontinued. This is akin to weeding the flowerbed and leaving the roots in; it gives an immediately gratifying appearance, but the end result is worse than at the beginning. In contrast, the indicated homeopathic remedy may initially aggravate the skin lesion, as if it is 'driving it out', yet the patient frequently says he 'feels better in himself'. Following this temporary aggravation, the condition usually slowly improves. This example is not implying that there is no place for topical steroids in treating eczema; they are indispensable when used correctly. I agree with Dr Margery Blackie, who was the homeopathic physician to H.M. Queen Elizabeth II for thirteen years, when she taught that eczema cannot be cured by homeopathy alone. Since its aetiology is multifactorial, effective treatment must include dealing with food intolerance, allergens (including house dust mite), sensitivity to washing powders, stress, and so on.

Homeopathic prescribing further differs from conventional prescribing in that only a single dose of the remedy is given, which is allowed to work until its action is exhausted. The patient has to heal himself – the dose merely initiates and stimulates that response. The second dose must be given only when the benefit from the first has worn off.

When a satellite is being put into orbit, the second and third stages of the rocket are fired only when the force of the thrust from the preceding stage has nearly ceased. The third stage usually puts the satellite into orbit. So too, in homeopathic prescribing, the secret of success is not to spoil the action of the medicine by over-frequent repetitions of the dose.

The benefit of one dose of some deep-acting remedies lasts for four to eight weeks, or longer. I have patients who have found that one dose of *Silica* in high potency will control their foot-sweat for six weeks or more. Moreover, when a homeopathic remedy eases a disorder it tends to cure it, rather than simply suppress symptoms, with the result that the need for giving further doses becomes progressively less frequent. I should add that in recent years I have prescribed potencies higher than 10M less often than before, as I am no longer convinced that they are more effective. I have also noticed that certain patients respond best to a certain potency in certain cases, for example, a woman with multiple allergies and atopic eczema found that *Sulphur* 30c was more beneficial than either *Sulphur* 6c or 200c.

Homeopathic potencies should not be repeated too soon, except in acute conditions. If the dose is repeated too soon an 'aggravation' may be provoked, which must be allowed to settle before any more doses are given. For example, I prescribed *Picric acid* 30c for a young man who complained of inability to concentrate, tired limbs and so on. As he felt so much better after the first dose, he helped himself – contrary to my instructions – twice daily. He got worse and worse, until on the fourth day he could hardly stand.

Similarly, a middle-aged woman had for ten years suffered from drenching night sweats, such that she had to change her nightdress several times a night. She was a chilly person, better in the open air, who could not tolerate fats and slept best late into the morning. I gave her *Pulsatilla* 200c, one dose, and she had her first good night for five months, only waking twice with the sweats. On succeeding nights she slept right through.

As she was due to return to London, I gave her a spare dose of *Pulsatilla* 200c, only to be taken when really indicated. Unfortunately, she repeated the dose far too soon and had her worst night for months. She contacted me and I gave her nothing, telling her that she could now expect weeks of freedom, which proved to be the case.

As you make a start yourself using homeopathic medicines, remember these basic principles, and do not be daunted by the apparent complexity of the case.

Chapter 3

First Aid

Homeopathy is often thought of as a gentle, slow-acting therapy, but in the treatment of emergencies, whether arising from accident, sudden illness or emotional trauma, it has a great deal to offer, much of which is unknown and unavailable to other disciplines.

GENERAL APPLICATIONS

Aconite

Aconite has been my best standby in acute medical emergencies. It is indicated in all cases of mental or physical shock or fright, with any of the following symptoms: tremor, palpitations, hyperventilation or gasping for breath; tight feeling in the chest; feeling cold or hot, collapse, or obvious fright or distress. Also eye injuries.

I met the aconite plant for the first time in 1975. I had seen many coloured pictures of it, and realised that to the uninitiated it looked like a purple snapdragon, although it is actually a delphinium. I knew too what the root should look like, as on numerous occasions it had caused fatalities when it had been wrongly identified as a horseradish. (A distinguishing feature is that the aconite root, when sectioned, turns red.) I had stopped by the roadside for a picnic on the way to 'La Grande Dixence' – the highest dam in Europe – and exploring a little stream that descended down the steep mountainside was suddenly aware of a strong smell of mint. Nearby was a patch of wild mint in which stood clumps of aconite in full bloom. I thought it unusual to find it here – it is an alpine plant, said to thrive on well-manured ground, normally found near to chalets, but there were neither cattle nor chalets in that remote part of Switzerland.

Aconite can boast an ancient and fascinating history, and has deservedly been called 'the Queen Mother of poisons' – it was also known as 'wolf's bane', and even as 'women's bane'! It was certainly an effective arrow poison. Plutarch relates that Orodes was cured of his dropsy by the juice of the plant: 'The dropsie received the poison, and the one drave the other out of Orodes' body and set him on foot again.' So the principle of homeopathy – 'let like be cured by like' or 'what a drug can cause it can cure' – was known to the Greeks. Hahnemann acknowledged that the ancients knew of this principle, and gives many examples in his *Organon*.

On a more macabre note, many years ago I came across the following cutting. I would like to pay tribute to the author who did this research, but the article was written anonymously:

Giving evidence on the detection of poisons in the body after death, Sir Robert Christison (1797–1882), professor of medical jurisprudence at Edinburgh University, stated that there was only one deadly agent which could not satisfactorily be traced, and that was ... when the judge interrupted him: 'Stop, please, Dr Christison. It is much better that the public should not know it.' It is interesting to know that the notorious Dr George Henry Lamson, who apparently was the first (1881) to employ aconitine with criminal intent, had attended Christison's lectures on toxicology as a medical student at Edinburgh. He thus knew that there was no chemical test for this substance and that it was unlikely to be recognised in post mortem. As it happened, a few words uttered by the dying victim referring to his 'throat closing', and his 'skin being drawn up', afforded a clue to Sir Thomas Stevenson, who identified the poison administered as being aconitine.

As a medical student my knowledge of *Aconite* was limited to its use as a liniment: 'Lin ABC' was very popular in those days. The three initials stood for *Aconite*, *Belladonna* and *Capsicum*. It is hardly ever used now. From a homeopathic point of view, a more useful triad of medicines is *Aconite, Belladonna* and *Calc. carb.* Potentised, these are frequently indicated in just that order in feverish conditions. For first aid home use you cannot go wrong by treating fever at its onset with *Aconite*. If after a few doses given frequently the condition deteriorates, follow on with *Belladonna* unless there are positive indications for an alternative homeopathic medicine, such as *Ferrum phos.* When the fever is all over, a dose of *Calc. carb.* may well be indicated, especially in the case of children, because this is the constitutional medicine for the clumsy, chubby, chilly, sweaty, constipated child – the very one to go down quickly with a high temperature when the wind is in the north-east. This is the weather that most calls for *Aconite* and *Belladonna*. (There are other 'East Wind Remedies', such as *Bryonia, Hepar sulph., Nux vomica* and *Spongia*, and any one of these may be required if the *Aconite* does not nip the illness in the bud.)

A father phoned at 11 a.m. about his five-year-old son who had vomited and had a temperature of 39.5°C (103°F). He was given *Aconite* 3x followed by *Belladonna* 6c. By 1.30 p.m. his temperature had dropped to 37.8°C (100°F), and by the evening he seemed completely well. Previously these attacks had been treated with antibiotics, and despite this the temperature would swing up and down for two days. A year later his mother, who was a senior administrator in the county's Children's Department, reported that for the first time he had not required any antibiotics for a year. 'The pills are marvellous.'

One way to remember the indications for *Aconite* is to take the words 'acute' and 'night', and join them to form a neologism, ACU-NIGHT. To be more accurate, transform this to ACU-FRIGHT, because these are the two states that cry out for the soothing influence of *Aconite*.

One morning I visited a local nursing home to see 92-year-old Mrs S., a new resident. The Matron told me that Mrs S. had arrived four days ago, but that she had not needed to send for me because she had been able to cope with her adequately. Apparently ten years previously Mrs S. had had a coronary. For the last year she had regularly been having nocturnal attacks of palpitation, which terrified her. She would call out for help, expecting another coronary, which could kill her. Unless someone came at once, and stayed two hours, she became increasingly breathless. In her restless state she would toss about, clutching her heart, begging for the window to be opened wider and pleading for help to get her head out of it for more air.

It was because of this distressing condition that her devoted family had reluctantly agreed to her admission, since they could endure their mother's plight and disturbed nights no longer. Predictably, the first night she had a typical attack. The night nurse was so concerned about her that she woke Matron. When Matron saw Mrs S., and I quote, 'I got that set of bottles with those sugar pills that you left for emergencies (Home Remedies), and found *Aconite*, which said 'for any emergency', and gave her one. It was marvellous; she settled down ever so quickly. I'm sure she simply panics and makes it worse for herself. I often use *Aconite* for different emergencies at night.'

Matron and I were discussing one of the other patients when a new care assistant came rushing in, white and trembling. (She herself was on my panel list, and I had known her from childhood.) 'Oh,' she burst out, 'I am sure Mrs H. has just died. I went in to see if she was all right, and when she didn't answer or move I touched her, and her head fell forward!' It was her first experience of death, and she was visibly shaking. I gave her an *Aconite* pill from my pocket case. Acute-Fright – very much so.

What then are the uses of *Aconite*? The label on the bottle supplied in the Home Remedy Kit reads:

ACONITE: SHOCK and No. 1 FEVER

For shock, croup, effects of fright or chills; any emergencies, e.g. accident, animal bites, asthma, haemorrhage, bereavement, distress, breathlessness, palpitations, tremblings, or numb tinglings. At onset of fevers, if thirsty, restless, anxious.

10 granules (one tablet or pill) every hour until relief

The Home Remedy Kit is issued as tablets (or granules in a few cases), normally in the 30c potency, unless a request is made for a different potency. I only carry and use a 10M potency of *Aconite* for cases where the mental changes are most pronounced, i.e. panic, shock, fright, etc.

An 18-year-old girl came with her mother to surgery. She complained of attacks of tingling in her arms and fingers. At the same time she felt dizzy and faint and was very conscious of her heart beating rapidly and forcefully. The mother volunteered: 'I used to get turns like that when I was her age.' I suspected that the girl was hyperventilating, although both she and her mother denied that this was so. In this state a person, usually when emotionally disturbed, takes rapid, shallow, panting breaths, with the result that they blow out their carbon dioxide and develop hypocapnia (it is a little more complicated than that) until ultimately they can actually go unconscious. Before this stage is reached they develop a plethora of different disconnected symptoms involving any system of the body.

The symptoms this girl had experienced were typical. Whatever the cause, I was safe in giving her *Aconite* for these attacks. It proved most effective. If the attacks persisted it would be necessary to enquire further into the cause of them and give a longer-acting medicine to prevent them.

Croup is another condition mentioned on the instruction label.

I received a phone call at 1 a.m. concerning a 3-year-old boy who could not get his breath and was very distressed, gasping and suffocating, with a loud, barking, croupy cough. The only medicine in the house was *Aconite*; I told them to give him a dose every fifteen minutes and put on a steam kettle, and to ring me after half an hour if he was no better.

The phone call came at morning surgery. After three doses he had gone to sleep, but had woken at 3 a.m. with another, less severe attack. *Aconite* was repeated, and in half an hour he was asleep again. Next morning he was as bright as a button.

If asked, 'In what type of illness or emergency do you use *Aconite*?', I might turn the question to 'When do I not use *Aconite*?', because I routinely use it on arrival at the scene of road accidents, coronary thrombosis, sudden death, burns, scalds, funerals – any and every occasion where panic, fright or shock are in evidence.

Arnica

If I were allowed to use only three homeopathic medicines, my choice would be *Arnica, Aconite* and *Belladonna*. *Arnica* is the medicine of first choice for bruises, sprains, contusions, head injuries, concussional headaches and myocardial infarction. It prevents and relieves muscle fatigue from overexertion.

Dosage

Use in any potency which is available: 6c, 30c, 200c or 10M, repeating every fifteen minutes in acute conditions, and otherwise every two to four hours. Locally it can be applied in a cream, or as a compress, provided that the skin is unbroken. For this purpose a solution is made from 2 to 3 ml of mother tincture (designated ø) in a cupful of cold water. *Arnica* in high potency is so effective when taken internally that local treatment is rarely necessary.

I was taking my daughter and her friend Sue (the daughter of a retired senior surgeon), home from a lacrosse match. On getting into my car my daughter slammed the front door, crushing Sue's left index finger. She cried out with pain, and I immediately gave her one pill of *Arnica* 10M from my pocket case. Ten minutes later I gave her a second dose. She said, 'The pain has already stopped, that pill is marvellous.' By now there was a slight subungual haematoma forming. I gave her six further doses to take at half-hourly intervals, and told her to tell her father it was homeopathic *Arnica*. I dropped her at the entrance of the drive leading to her house a quarter of an hour later, and she said her finger was not hurting.

Feeling some guilt, and still being concerned about her, I phoned her father that evening, and before I could apologise he said, 'Whatever is in those pills? My daughter is most impressed, and is emphatic that her finger does not hurt. I have looked up the word *Arnica* in all my books,

24

and cannot find anything about it, but Sue insists I buy a bottle of these pills. Where can I get them?' I told him a little about homeopathy, and he kept repeating, 'She is most impressed, and so am I.'

I issued *Arnica* in the 30th potency to each family I treated, with the instructions:

ARNICA: INJURY

For bruises, sprains, concussion, crushed fingers, road accidents, etc. If shocked, give *Aconite* first. Also for exhaustion or muscle aching (heart, chest, back or limbs) from strain, sport or overuse. Use before or after dental surgery.

10 granules (one tablet or pill) every two hours until relief

If there were room on the label, it could usefully include: 'As first-aid for coronary thrombosis'.

In one surgery session I prescribed *Arnica* six times, to:

1) A sixteen-year-old girl with a bruised chin following a fall from her horse.
2) A housewife who had sprained her thumb when trying to open a sardine tin.
3) A man who had a concrete slab fall onto his shins.
4) A foundry worker complaining of an aching back and legs, after his first week of work in his new job.
5) A schoolboy with a sprained forefoot.
6) A keen soccer player who had stubbed his toes against the goal-post – and hadn't even scored a goal as a compensation!

I had been using this most useful remedy on an average of once a day for about twenty years before I ever saw an arnica plant, or even a good coloured illustration of one. (It is not in Culpeper's *Herbal*.) I was at Martigny, in Switzerland, on my way to the Furka Pass, when I saw an illustrated packet of arnica seeds in a shop window. Some hours later I stopped near the top of the pass to enjoy the scenery. By now I was over 1500 m (5000 ft) high but still there was an abundance of conifers, larches and stone pines growing on the mountain side. I could see snow-capped mountain peaks standing up against the clear blue sky away in the distance. It was here that I discovered my first arnica flowers. They stood up nearly ten feet tall, with large orange-yellow flower heads. I would have liked to pick one, but contented myself with photographing them instead. On the way down the pass I found some more plants growing near the roadside on the sparsely-covered rocks. They were in a very exposed, windswept position.

Later I found a chemist in Lausanne who sold packets of arnica leaves, with a vivid-coloured picture of the flower on the label. On the reverse side there were instructions in German and French for making both a compress and a medicine for internal use to treat bruises and dislocations. I have heard Dr Blackie say that the Swiss guides take arnica at the beginning of each season to prevent muscle soreness after their first climb.

Aconite and *Arnica* between them probably are indicated in 80% of all accidents and emergencies, and many doctors have been converted to homeopathy following their initial experiments and successes with these two remedies. Often they are all that is needed, and the patient's own homeostatic response will complete the healing; in other cases different remedies may be required to complete the cure.

Calendula (Marigold)

For cuts, lacerations, abrasions, gravel rash, burns, sore fissures and bed sores. Used as a mouthwash it is an excellent haemostatic after dental extraction. Also valuable externally after episiotomy.

Dosage

Use internally in potency 12c to 200c, or apply locally in aqueous solution (5 ml to 500 ml or 10 drops of tincture to half a pint of water), oil, cream or ointment.

Carbo vegetabilis (Vegetable Charcoal)

For collapse or faint. A valuable remedy in vasovagal attacks or in more severe collapse, post-operatively or in cardiac cases, where the patient is cold, bluish, sweaty, with cold extremities, thin thready pulse, and a desire for air at a window, or to be fanned.

Dosage

30c to 10M potency given frequently, either in granules dry on the tongue or in water, every five to ten minutes until response, and then at longer intervals.

Hypericum (St John's Wort)

For nerve injuries – as in crushed fingertips, painful animal bites (dogs, cats, rodents, etc.), penetrating puncture wounds such as from splinters, thorns and nails. Post-operative pain. Lacerations.

St John's Wort, like marigold, is another plant quoted by Culpeper in his *Herbal,* and for centuries has been used to relieve painful injuries to soft parts richly supplied with nerve endings. In the case of a crushed fingertip, it would be indicated if the pain persisted. (*Arnica* is given first, to stop the extravasation of blood beneath the nail.) The homeopathic use of St John's Wort is not to be confused with its use herbally (i.e. in material doses) to treat depression.

Dosage

As for *Calendula. Hypercal* ointment, containing *Hypericum* and *Calendula*, is both soothing and healing.

Ledum (Mash Tea)

The chief remedy for puncture wounds, for example a nail into the sole of the foot. Also of value in bruising around the eye, where it seems to be even better than *Arnica*. The pains of *Ledum* are always worse from heat, and better for local cold applications.

Dosage

30c to 10M potency, repeated every two to four hours as required. In deep, potentially septic wounds, tetanus immunisation should also be given.

Rhus toxicodendron (Poison Ivy)

The poison ivy, in potency, is indicated for the effects of strains where the muscle stiffness and aching are temporarily relieved by movement, are worse at rest, and are worst after prolonged rest. The first movements to 'limber up' after a night's sleep are the most painful.

Dosage

30c to 10M potency, every two hours.

Ruta (Rue)

Ruta is ideal for treating strains of ligaments around joints, when the symptoms are 'like *Rhus tox.*, but more so'. Particularly where periosteal attachments are involved.

Dosage

30c potency, every two to four hours. Both *Ruta* and *Rhus tox.* can follow *Arnica*.

Staphysagria (Stavesacre)

Useful in incised wounds, and therefore after operation, especially in gynaecological repairs. It relieves pain and helps healing.

Dosage

30c to 10M potency, repeated every two hours for six doses.

Symphytum (Comfrey or Knitbone)

Used in lowest potencies (3x to 6x) *Symphytum* has the reputation of accelerating the union of fractures, and is also very useful in treating contusions of the eye.

HEAD INJURIES

Where drowsiness persists despite medication with *Arnica*, give *Opium* 30c upwards, and if there is still no improvement consider the need for *Helleborus*. It is assumed that the practitioner would admit the patient to a neurological unit for observation, should his condition warrant it.

For persistent post-concussional headaches unrelieved by *Arnica*, use *Natrum sulph.* 30c.

INSECT AND PLANT STINGS

Homeopathy certainly has more to offer than the old-fashioned treatments with blue-bag, vinegar or lemon juice, and offers a satisfactory alternative to the conventional treatment with topical steroids and antihistamines.

Traditionally, *Ledum* (Marsh Tea) is given in low potency for bee and wasp stings, when the sting or bite is relieved by cold applications. I prefer to give *Apis mellifica* (potentised honey-bee) to victims of bee stings, and *Vespa vulgaris* (wasp) to those stung by wasps. In both cases low potencies should be used, repeated every five minutes until relief. Kent lists remedies for stings under 'Skins'. Animal bites are given under 'Wounds' in Generalities.

As a local application, a compress of *Urtica urens* is very soothing, as is *Hypercal* ointment.

Urtica urens (Stinging Nettle)

The nettle is effective used internally in potency, and externally as a compress, for nettle stings and any allergic urticarial reactions that simulate nettle stings, provided the skin is intact.

Cantharis (Spanish Fly)

Spanish fly in 30c potency is effective in treating gnat bites, where painful blisters result which burn when touched, and where the affected skin rapidly necroses. *Pyrethrum* liquid is a useful deterrent against gnat bites, and should be diluted and applied to the exposed parts of the skin.

BURNS

Both *Urtica* and *Cantharis* cause and cure burning vesication of the skin, and accordingly are used in the homeopathic treatment of burns. They are applied in the form of ointments and creams, or *Urtica* lotion (5 ml to 500 ml or 10 drops to one pint of boiled water) and may also be given internally in the 30c potency every fifteen minutes to two hours, according to the severity of the symptoms, until relief.

I quote the personal experience of a colleague: 'Inadvertently I grasped a casserole which had just been taken out of an oven heated to 200°C (390°F). I felt a searing pain, and an angry, dark red weal appeared across the palmar surfaces of four fingers. I quickly applied *Urtica urens* cream (always at hand in the kitchen) and took a tablet of *Urtica urens* 30c. The pain abated within minutes, and about six hours later all redness had faded and I was able to use the hand normally. The incident was forgotten until several days later, when a layer of skin peeled off the burned area, leaving it clean and healthy.'

HEATSTROKE

Belladonna (Deadly Nightshade)

This is an excellent remedy for the effects of sun exposure, and rapidly controls the fever, headache and malaise. If the headache persists, use *Glonoine*.

CHILLING

Camphor

An excellent prophylactic against the effects of being chilled, and as such is most useful for doctors who have to do night visits. A dose taken every five minutes until warmed will usually prevent a cold or diarrhoea from developing. If taken at the onset, *Camphor* will abort an attack of diarrhoea, if the patient feels very cold.

It is interesting to note that *Camphor* was one of Hahnemann's specifics for the treatment of cholera.

Chapter 4

Mental Illness

The Importance of Mental Symptoms in Choosing the Remedy

Homeopathic prescribing is not easy, because the remedy of choice must match the patient as much as the illness that is being treated. In other words, the prescription must be 'tailor made' rather than 'off the peg'. As a result of this it often happens that, in treating several consecutive cases of a particular illness, one has to use a different remedy for each patient. This is because the remedy that is indicated for the first patient would be quite unsuited for the others, and therefore would be ineffective.

Over the course of years it becomes possible to associate certain people with certain homeopathic medicines, because they match so well. Consequently, the same medicine may be indicated for that particular person for quite a variety of illnesses. This should not surprise us when we consider that, in using homeopathy, we are trying to restore health by stimulating the homeostatic responses of the patient, rather than by suppressing various disease symptoms. Although the disease to be treated may manifest itself in different organs and systems of the body, and in various ways, health will only be fully restored when the body can be encouraged to heal itself, and the indicated homeopathic medicine will do this.

DEPRESSION

As an illustration of this, let me cite the diverse symptoms of depression. This frequently presents with general symptoms such as lassitude, loss of appetite, insomnia, breathlessness, loss of interest and energy, even before the more florid feelings of depression, failure, guilt and unworthiness emerge. Hahnemann taught that there were illnesses that were brought on by depression, grief, anger, resentment, etc., and he listed appropriate medicines for such, despite the protean patterns of symptoms that characterised the illness. This is why, in

31

prescribing, he insisted one must give greatest prominence to the 'mental' symptoms, then the 'generals' and finally the 'particulars', in that order.

By 'mentals' he meant any variation from the normal in feelings or mood (affect). Leaving depression aside, let us look at the features of an anxiety state. If, as happens all too frequently these days, a person is under prolonged stress due to some insoluble domestic or marital problem, it is not surprising that, in time, some system of the body reacts unfavourably, or even breaks down. The symptoms that may be present are legion, including sweating, tension headaches or backache, colic, palpitations and breathlessness.

The experienced doctor will enquire or even probe into causative social or environmental factors which could have precipitated (or could be perpetuating) these complaints. Having explored the feelings of the patient and discovered the 'heartaches and headaches' that were being silently endured, he might point out that the patient was not really 'suffering in silence', as he thought, but that some parts of the body were literally suffering, and crying out in protest.

The homeopath would then look for an indicated medicine among the 'Mind' section of his repertory. He would not start looking for the remedy in the various sections dealing with individual symptoms such as:

1) Head – pain (headaches)
2) Perspiration
3) Chest – palpitations
4) Abdomen – colic

because the number of likely remedies to choose from would run into hundreds. Bear in mind that most drugs in toxic doses will cause a headache, so that in Kent's *Repertory* we find eighty-five pages of detail about remedies that can cause, and therefore cure, headaches! Instead, we must look for them in the 'Mind' section of the repertory, for example: 'Mind: Anger, ailments after'. In this way we can take a shortcut and find the answer in much less time.

The remedies which particularly suit ailments from the following emotions are:

1) Anger – *Aconite, Chamomilla, Cocculus, Colocynthis, Ignatia, Ipecacuanha, Nux vomica, Opium, Platina, Staphysagria*
2) Indignation – *Staphysagria*
3) Grief – *Aurum, Causticum, Cocculus, Ignatia, Lachesis, Natrum mur., Phosphoric acid, Staphysagria*

4) Jealousy – *Lachesis*
5) Reproach – *Opium*
6) Rudeness – *Staphysagria*

I have listed only those printed in the repertory in heavy black type, which therefore most prominently display these 'mentals'.

Admittedly one may have to turn to the appropriate sections of the repertory to confirm my findings, and look for 'Backache from anger', 'Colic from anger', but the mental clue has been invaluable. Backache caused by anger does not appear to be listed, but colic caused by anger becomes a 'strange, rare or peculiar' symptom, only found under a few remedies (*Chamomilla*, *Colocynth*, *Nux vomica*, *Staphysagria* and *Sulphur*). This whittles down the list of possibly indicated remedies to just five, which is an extremely useful shortcut.

General and Particular Symptoms

By 'generals' Hahnemann meant general symptoms that affected the whole person, rather than an individual part. Thus 'I am feeling very chilly' is a general symptom, and in a person who normally is 'warm-blooded' and never feels the cold, would be a very significant symptom. It would point to such remedies as *Arsenicum album* and *Nux vomica*.

'Particulars' in contrast, are symptoms referable to a localised part of the body, which are described as 'My left arm is tingling' or 'My head is throbbing'. If now a person has both the 'general' 'Feeling very cold and chilly' and wants to be wrapped up warmly even in a warm room, and yet has the paradoxical 'particular' 'Hot, burning, throbbing headache' which is eased by getting his head into cold air, or by cold applications, then this would make one think of *Arsenicum album*: 'Blankets up to the chin and head out of the window'. If, as well, the patient were feeling very anxious and fearful, weak and restless, and had a thirst for little sips of warm water, then the choice of *Arsenicum album* would be confirmed. But remember – of all those indications listed, the mentals 'Fearful and anxious and mentally restless' are more important than all the others.

ANXIETY

Another example is the case of a person who has just had a very severe fright.

The physiological response one would expect would be for the person to feel cold, for the heart to start beating forcibly and fast (palpitations), the mouth to go dry, the skin to perspire a sense of constriction to develop in the chest, followed by a feeling of suffocation or faintness. All these somatic (bodily) symptoms are due to the fright that affected the mind in the first place.

In the 'Mind' section of the repertory, under the heading of 'Fright; complaints from', we find *Aconite* listed among the nine medicines in heavy bold black type. It would be a laborious task to try to repertorise by searching under the several headings 'Palpitations', 'Dry mouth', 'Perspiration' etc. Those are all 'particulars' of lesser rank than the 'mentals', which must take pride of place.

The 'general' symptom 'Feeling cold' comes next, and again we find *Aconite* prominent in the section 'Heat, vital, lack of'. Until the fright is removed and the mind calmed, the adrenal glands will continue to pour out adrenaline into the bloodstream, and all the 'particular' symptoms will persist. Tranquillise the mind, and the rest of the body will become calm in sympathy.

This is why, to an almost alarming degree, tranquillisers are being prescribed increasingly to combat the distressing bodily disorders that follow emotional upsets. The use of homeopathy can avoid such drugs to a large extent.

MIND AND MATTER

The fact that significant mood changes occur in physical illness has long been recognised by doctors practising homeopathy. Indeed, the fact that Kent, following Hahnemann's teaching, gives 'mentals' pride of place among the prescribing features of disease shows he was a century ahead of his conventional colleagues. It had always been accepted that in jaundice the person became melancholic; indeed, the derivation of the word suggests this. Similarly, people suffering from gout become unbearably rude and irritable, and in contrast, terminal cases of tuberculosis displayed an unusual degree of euphoria. But beyond a few isolated examples such as these, medical practitioners failed to recognise, or ignored, the alterations in the affect, volition, memory or comprehension of their sick patients.

In the same way, time-aggravation symptoms that have become priceless prescribing clues to the homeopathically–orientated practitioner were overlooked or counted of no value by their 'orthodox' colleagues. Research workers in the field of psychiatry have explored these subjects, determining the possibility of biochemical variations in the body causing mental ill-health, and studied the disturbances of diurnal rhythm in people suffering from depression.

It is known that the cortisol levels in the body follow a diurnal rhythm, accounting for periods of low arousal, as during the early hours of the morning and in the early afternoon. This rhythm is disturbed by various illnesses, such as endogenous depression, in which early morning awakening is seen. Light affects melatonin levels, causing hibernation in some animals when the day shortens. Melatonin is produced by the pineal gland, which was thought to be vestigial in humans but is now known to be important, and produces the changes in sleep patterns seen in, for example, jet lag.

These observations immediately throw light on the fascinating alterations of mood and thought content that Hahnemann noted and recorded so carefully in his original remedy provings, and also on the question of time aggravations. It is likely that these changes in turn are precipitated and controlled by biochemical variations in the body, from which it can follow that the administration of the required medicine can restore the balance, with resultant return to mental and physical health. They may indicate that, in the same way that lithium carbonate in material doses can control many cases of manic depression, metallic gold in potency (*Aurum metallicum*) can alleviate depression, and potentised *Sepia* remove feelings of hostility towards loved ones.

Again, in a slightly different context, one of Freud's earliest and most brilliant pupils, Theodor Reik, taught: 'Most problems of sexual incompatibility can be solved if the analyst approaches them as possible manifestations of unconscious resentment and hurt pride.' (*Psychology of Sex Relations*). This agrees with homeopathic thinking, explaining why *Platina* can help in such situations, probably just as effectively and far more quickly than the lengthy psychoanalysis he advocated. Among the provings of *Platina* we find not only 'haughty', 'arrogant', 'proud', under mentals, but also (under particulars) 'aversion to coition' (p.715, Kent). For the same remedy, under mentals, we find 'nymphomania' in prominent type, confirming that feelings can swing violently. So too, under the mental symptom 'Ailments from anger' (Kent, p.2) both *Natrum mur.* and *Staphysagria* are in prominent type. Both, too, are associated with aversion to sexual relations (Kent, p.715).

What modern psychiatrists now tacitly accept was propounded by Hahnemann over a century ago.

The following two cases describe physical illness associated with or, more probably, resulting from, mental disturbances. The details of the homeopathic prescribing are presented in full for the first case only. The remedy in each case was worked out mainly on 'mentals' and 'generals' alone. Where it was possible to establish a positive thermal reaction (aggravation to heat or cold) of the patient as a whole, then either all the 'hot' or all the 'cold' remedies were eliminated from each rubric.

CASE 1

George was a cheerful, overactive, blue-eyed, stocky boy of four, whom I knew very well. He came of a closely-knit family, and his parents were well adjusted.

He came on our annual Sunday School outing to Blackpool in July 1964, and strayed, and was separated from his parents for about twenty minutes. (Apparently he had climbed some steps, keeping his parents in sight; and a well-meaning woman had assumed he was lost and forcibly taken him to the Lost Children's Crèche, despite his protests.) By the time he was reunited with his parents he was very distressed, and within a few days a perceptible mood change developed.

This change was first described to me on 19 August. If denied anything, or corrected, he would cry loudly and stamp his feet, or shake his arm in temper; he could not be left alone, especially at night, and he had anorexia. I gave him *Cina* 200c (see Boericke) and chloral hydrate elixir.

My assistant saw him two weeks later and prescribed a double dose of phenobarbitone elixir, as the child was now very frightened of the dark and of being alone.

On 25 November he was brought to see me again, because 'things were getting desperate'. His mother reported that no matter how early he was put to bed, he would not drop off to sleep before 10 p.m., and he would wake regularly at 1.30 a.m., 3 a.m., and 5 a.m., when he would get up for the day (or lie awake until permission to do so was given). During the night he insisted on having the light on, and even insisted that the landing light be left on and his bedroom door left open. In short, he was terrified of the dark. In addition, he was afraid of travelling.

His behaviour and mood I summarised thus:

He was tearful – his tears were uncontrollable when rebuked. He was obstinate and sullen.

He had visual and auditory hallucinations, 'seeing little black men and hearing voices' (Kent 'Delusions: images, phantoms, sees, black').

He was afraid of the dark and of being alone, but was not upset by thunder. He had anorexia, but had developed a craving for sugar and sweets. Whereas before he would have carried a packet of sweets in his pocket for a week, now he would eat the entire contents in one morning. Nothing tasted sweet enough. Prior to this illness he had not liked sweet things but had preferred salty foods and sauces.

He had a thirst for cold drinks, wanting even his tea and coffee cold; this too was a reversal of his previous likes.

He suffered from insomnia, inasmuch as he woke regularly.

I noted his physical appearance, and the fact that his pupils were fully dilated. There was no marked reaction to heat or cold, but if anything he was slightly 'cold-blooded'.

After repertorising, I gave him *Stramonium* 30c (thorn-apple), one tablet, to be repeated each morning following a badly disturbed night.

Ten days later his mother reported a great improvement from the first night. She had not had to use any sedative elixir but had had to give him a dose of *Stramonium* on alternate mornings for three doses, and every third morning since. The boy was sleeping better, only waking once during the night, at about 1.30 a.m. He was less nervous, and his pupils were now not markedly dilated. I gave him *Stramonium* 200c with the same instructions as before.

Three weeks later, on 30 December, I saw him again, when the mother reported that she had had to give him a dose almost every second morning, and that if she withheld this he would wake once and ask for the light to be put on. They were able to leave his light on only till he fell asleep, and with his regular medication he slept right through each night. He no longer had tantrums when thwarted and had stopped asking for sugar, having reverted to his old preference for tomato sauce.

He remained well without medication until 20 August 1965, when his symptoms returned following his spending a weekend with his aunt. The picture was identical: night terrors, fear of the dark, fear of being alone, pupils dilated, and preference for sweets. In error, I gave him *Hyoscyamus* 12c (henbane) and the mother returned a week later, surprised at having no improvement to report. I gave *Stramonium* 30c, and the symptoms once again quickly subsided.

In the autumn of 1967 the family left the district, but a year later an aunt, who visited them regularly, said that George 'never looked back'.

Analysis of the Case

Repertorising was complicated by the fact that the boy had no pronounced temperature reactions, so it was not possible, in each rubric, to eliminate either the 'hot' or 'cold' medicines. Taking the most unusual mental alterations in order (using Kent's *Repertory*) we have:

1) Fear of the dark: Twenty-two medicines listed, only two in heavy black type, i.e. CAN. IND., STRAM.; and *Phos.* and *Lyc.* in italics.
2) Fear of being alone: Forty-three medicines listed, seven in heavy black type, i.e. ARG.NIT., ARS., CROT. C., HYOS., KALI C., PHOS., LYC.; *Stram.* in italics.
3) Visual hallucinations: Delusions: sees images, faces, men, black. Seventy medicines, only BELL. and LACHESIS in heavy black type, seventeen in italics, including *Stram.*
4) Auditory hallucinations: Delusions: voices, hears. No large black type medicines. Six in italics including *Phos.*, and *Lyc.* and *Stram.* in small type.

Then, under various particulars, we have – in order of urgency and peculiar significance:

5) Sleep interrupted: Fifty medicines, none in heavy type. Two only in italics: *Alum.*, and *Stram.*; *Lyc.*, and *Phos.* small type.
6) Pupils dilated: A hundred and one remedies, nine in heavy black type: ARG. NIT., BELL., CALC., CHIN., GELS., HYOS., MANG., SEC., STRAM. *Phos.* in italics. *Lyc.* in small type.
7) Desires sweets: p.486. Thirty-six medicines, four in heavy type: ARG. NIT., CHIN., LYC., SULPH.

If we now score 3 for bold type, 2 for italics and 1 for plain type, we get the unequivocal result: *Arg. Nit.* 9; *Lyc.* 11; *Phos.* 10; *Stram.* 14. If, however, we had confined our repertorising to the strong, distinctive mental symptoms (which, in fact, disturbed the patient and distressed the parents) and had included sleep disturbance because this was inseparably linked with it, the results would have been just as clear-cut: *Arg. Nit.*, 3; *Lyc.* 7; *Phos.* 8; *Stram.* 11. Of these four remedies only *Lyc.* has a heat aggravation, and *Stramonium* is associated with the most florid mental disturbances. As results show, it was the remedy of choice.

An undesigned confirmation that *Stramonium* was the right remedy was the failure to improve again, after the inadvertent administration of *Hyoscyamus* in August 1965, which the parents presumed to be the same medicine as before.

When the indicated remedy, *Stramonium*, was prescribed, immediate benefit followed. Consider, too, the fact that the two popular and potent conventional sedatives (chloral hydrate and phenobarbitone) given in maximum doses, plus incorrectly prescribed homeopathic remedies (*Cina* and *Hyos.*) failed to help before the indicated homeopathic medicine was discovered and given.

This answers the possible criticism that the boy recovered only because it was the parents who needed reassurance and help, and that once that had been afforded, even a placebo would have achieved the same results. Many child psychiatrists feel that most behaviour problems in children under four years old are really parent problems, i.e. an expression of, or a result from, conflicts between the parents; or they are parent-child problems.

This case illustrates the need to give preference to the extraordinary mental symptoms, which, when marked, must dominate the case.

CASE 2

Hazel was a small, thin 4½-year-old girl, with fair skin and hair. She had always been a very shy, retiring girl, hiding behind her mother's skirts whenever I saw her or even spoke to her in the street. She was very difficult to please and was fussy about her food. As an only child (by design), she had always been spoiled by her well-meaning and over-indulgent parents and grandparents.

On 25.1.65 her mother attended, seeking help. She reported that over the past year Hazel had been becoming aggressive, but that in the last few months she had got completely out of hand. 'She has always had a bit of temper, even as a baby, but recently she has been having mad fits. She has temper tantrums when she will shake with rage, and maliciously kick and punch me.' She further stated that Hazel had become hypersensitive to noise, putting her fingers into her ears. The tantrums were uncontrolled by correction (at least by the modified form administered by her mother).

I gave six pilules of *Staphysagria* 12c, with instructions to give one twice a day until reaction.

Only two doses were needed. Hazel's mother later reported, 'She has not had a tantrum since the first dose; usually she had at least one an evening.' *Staphysagria* was prescribed on the prominent mental change that had transformed a shy, retiring, chilly child into an oversensitive one, evidencing violent outbursts of passion.

I confess to giving it virtually on this one dominant mental indication, as the surgery was crowded that winter morning and I had no time to collect further details. I appreciated that if my choice of remedy were incorrect, the mother inevitably would return and I would have to prescribe more accurately. I was as gratified as the parents to find how successful the therapy proved to be.

The cure could hardly be attributed to coincidental spontaneous recovery. In my experience in similar situations, matters, if untreated, tend to deteriorate rather than improve. Equally, it is not a valid criticism to suggest that the improvement followed some form of psychotherapy, because the first interview lasted only about three minutes.

These two case histories illustrate how disabling physical illnesses of emotionally induced origin can be significantly improved by giving the homeopathic simillimum.

MEMORY LOSS

CASE 3

Arthur, aged 66, had become very forgetful following a stroke nine months previously. He attended on 28.10.71 complaining of floaters in his eyes. As he was leaving the surgery, his daughter (who had brought him) said, 'By the way, can you do anything for Dad's memory? He can't remember a thing these days.' The patient confirmed this.

As a 'shot in the dark' I gave him one dose of *Anacardium orientale* (marking nut) 200c; and thought no more about it, as they were both due to leave the district in the next couple of weeks.

On 17.11.71 the daughter phoned and said there had been a most dramatic improvement in her father's memory within two days of the medication. She and her husband just could not account for it, and thought it was almost 'spooky'. The patient himself was delighted, as he could now remember things he had long since forgotten.

At this stage I cautiously asked the daughter whether her father tended to be irascible and use unsuitable language, and she said, 'Well, yes, surprisingly; when he had been getting irritable on account of his. memory loss, he had been cursing and swearing, which was completely out of character.' I agreed she could collect three spare doses, only to be used when necessary, probably at intervals of two to three months.

I noticed that my supply of *Anacardium* 200c was dated 13 September 1949, which confirms the fact that homeopathic medicines, made by a reputable pharmacy, seem to keep their strength virtually indefinitely, if kept in a cool place away from strong odours.

Interestingly, he had no symptoms of dyspepsia, or amelioration from food, which one might have expected, as these features are present in the materia medica of *Anacardium*.

CASE 4

On 17.1.74 a 78-year-old widow, who had been on my panel list since the inception of the NHS in 1948, was brought to morning surgery by one of her daughters, who complained of her mother's hopeless memory. 'She can't remember a thing; she prepares potatoes for roasting, and then starts boiling them. She gets so confused, forgets what she is doing, and what she did a few hours before.'

I gave her five tablets of *Anacardium* 200c, three to be given that day in separate doses, and two spare doses to be taken at fortnightly intervals.

They returned a month later when the daughter reported a great improvement:

'Before we came to you she would say "What time of day is it? Is it Sunday?" (when it was Tuesday), and kept on like that ... we've had none of that since.'

When I asked what she thought had made the improvement she replied: 'Those memory tablets. Before she had them she was really down, but after taking the first one she picked up in two days and was as right as rain. You said we had to give one every fortnight, and when the next one was nearly due she started going back again. But after each memory tablet she picked up again, and that's why I've come for some more.'

PARANOIA

CASE 5

A 40-year-old plasterer suddenly became suspicious of his wife's fidelity, returning home from work at all hours of the day to check what she was doing.

She had to get his permission before walking to the village shops, and when they went dancing together she had learned never to dance with anyone else but him.

At times he became hypomanic. All this was totally out of character.

In July 1974 I gave the wife some granules of *Hyoscyamus* 10M to lace his tea unobtrusively, one dose to be administered as required at approximately two-week intervals. I warned her that if he spotted what she was doing and accused her of poisoning him, she must bring me into it, tell him it was my instruction, and contact me immediately if he became agitated or aggressive.

Two weeks later she reported a very great improvement, but found it necessary to continue giving fortnightly doses for the next five months.

Hahnemann quoted many examples of effective therapies used by the medical authorities of his day that were based on the homeopathic principle, including the use of hyoscyamus in treating mania; before the advent of phenothiazines it was the treatment of choice in our mental hospitals. Yet an overdose of henbane makes a person suspicious, fearful, jealous and paranoid.

Larger doses produce confusion, acute mania and even acute delirium.

I am not a psychiatrist, but did work at one of Birmingham's largest mental hospitals for twenty-two years as a clinical assistant. I would never rely on homeopathic medicines alone to treat acute psychosis, but they can indeed be a very useful adjunct.

Chapter 5

Neurological Disease

In homeopathic terms, neurological disease presents perhaps the greatest challenge. Many diseases are untreatable conventionally, and relentlessly progressive. Homeopathy does not by any means claim to cure them but, in terms of quality of life, symptom relief can contribute a huge benefit.

A range of clinical conditions are presented below, with discussion of some lesser-used medicines in some cases. Finally, the much more commonplace problems of migraine and headaches are included, which all practitioners will have to treat frequently.

TUBEROUS SCLEROSIS

CASE 6

Tuberous Sclerosis (TS) is a rare but well-recognised hereditary neuro-ectodermal disease, first clearly described in 1880, and also known as epiloia. Although dominantly inherited, over 50% of patients represent new mutations. Pathologically there are malformations or tumours of many organs, especially of the skin and CNS. Its features include:

1) Mental retardation, in 60% of cases,
2) Epilepsy, in 80% of cases,
3) Skin lesions: most commonly a disfiguring acne-like rash (adenoma sebaceum) in a butterfly distribution on the face. In infants there may be hypopigmentation of the skin (mountain ash leaf macules).

The Tuberous Sclerosis Association of Great Britain represents several hundred families where one or more members suffer from this disease. Whereas twenty years ago the incidence of TS in the population was estimated as 1:200,000 people, it is now thought to be as high as 1:20,000. This is presumed to be because better means of diagnosis (including CAT and MRI scanning) are now available.

43

The patient was a two-year-old boy who developed infantile spasms when five months old. In these attacks he suddenly, apparently spontaneously, would look vacant, his pupils dilate, and his face go pale. His right arm would twitch a few times, then, flexing at the waist, he bent double, finally falling onto the crown of his head. These are known as 'salaam spasms'. He would lie there, with eyes wide open, deviating to the left. His right arm would straighten, and repeatedly be elevated from his body and returned to his side again. There was no incontinence nor tongue biting. The attacks lasted from a half to one minute and his mother felt that he was conscious throughout, and could appreciate sound. The parents meticulously recorded the number of the attacks, which averaged between five or six each day and as many each night.

On 18 August 1986, at his first consultation, he presented as a cheerful lad, with a few scattered patches of under-pigmentation of the skin. He had been fully investigated at the Children's Hospital and was thought to be slightly mentally handicapped. He had right-sided weakness, especially of his right arm, which tended to hang limply by his side 'as if broken'. He was very unsteady on his feet. He was often irritable, and impatient. and was awake most nights until 4.30 a.m. His parents got more sleep if his mother slept beside him. His maintenance medication was sodium valproate 600 mg per day and nitrazepam 10 mg per day, both in divided doses. His mother was already using *Arnica* freely for his many falls.

18.8.86. I prescribed *Nux vomica* 6c (poison nut) four times a day. The sodium valproate and nitrazepam were continued. The *Nux vomica* was to be replaced with *Artemisia vulgaris* 3c (mugwort, wormwood) three times a day if there was no improvement in one week.

8.9.86. There had been no significant change with *Nux vomica* but slight but significant improvement on *Artemisia* 3c ('or is it coincidence?').

He had a fit during the consultation, which I witnessed. Experimentally I increased the potency of the *Artemisia* to 12c twice a day for a week, to be continued until reaction, then stop and wait. If no significant response after one week he was to be changed to *Cicuta* 3c four times a day for a week, and if still no response replaced with *Oenanthe crocata* 3c (water dropwort) three times a day.

20.10.86. No significant change with either *Cicuta* or *Oenanthe*, but some improvement on *Artemisia*. 'He is not dropping so much to the floor.' With the hospital's consent the parents had started slowly to reduce the nitrazepam and by now had halved his original daily dose to 5 mg daily in divided doses. The boy had recently become very hungry, with a voracious appetite, and was kicking off the bedclothes at night.

Treatment

> *Tuberculinum* 10M, one dose
> *Artemisia* 30c every 72 hours
> Continue sodium valproate

5.1.87. 'He seemed better the day after taking *Artemisia* 30c.'

The nitrazepam had been finally withdrawn by 8.11.86. The parents also tried withholding *Artemisia*, but after three weeks steady deterioration they resumed giving *Artemisia* 30c, and after the first dose he went four days without a single fit. He was now being given *Artemisia* 30c on alternate days as the parents found this controlled him better. The fits were milder and were only two a day on average. Sodium valproate 600 mg daily was continued, with *Artemisia* 30c when necessary.

22.1.87. Parents decided independently to do a trial of withholding *Artemisia* completely.

16.2.87. No increase in frequency of fits – still only two a day, and none by night, whereas eight months ago he had ten to twelve every 24 hours. Still taking sodium valproate.

7.3.87. In the last few weeks no drop attacks; most unusual. Parents very pleased. No *Artemisia* for six weeks.

13.6.87. 'Very well. Approximately two absences a day, for seconds only. No salaam attacks or fits for three months. Twice he has had a 'drop attack' landing on his bottom. He walks much more steadily and can even run and kick a football without falling over. He is learning to jump now. His right arm doesn't hang limply at his side – he now uses it to play, and reaches out with it to pick things up. Mentally he is developing better and attends a day nursery three times a week. He sleeps soundly from 8.30 p.m. to 8.30 a.m.! We had never believed it possible for him to sleep undisturbed right through the night. We don't think it is just normal development with age, because it all has happened so quickly.'

His mother had been giving him courses of *Artemisia* 30c on alternate days, for about a week, every few weeks when she had a feeling he was about to relapse.

45

Discussion

An isolated case history proves nothing, but it can be informative and might stimulate others to try homeopathic treatment in attempting to control this very distressing disease, which so often resists conventional medication. Frequently the dose of anticonvulsants that is necessary to control the fits profoundly disturbs the patient, to such a degree that the drug has to be withheld. Mental handicap is intensified by poor fit control and by excessive use of depressant anticonvulsants such as phenobarbitone and primidone. Poor fit control leads to a progressive loss of skills. Spontaneous remissions in infancy do occur, but apparently are unusual.

This case is interesting because three other homeopathic medicines known to be useful in treating convulsions were tried, without any subsequent change in the boy's condition. They were:

Nux vomica 3c (which contains strychnine)
Cicuta virosa 3c (which contains the poisonous alkaloid cicutine)
Oenanthe crocata 3c (in the same family as *Cicuta*)

It is not surprising that neither *Cicuta* nor *Oenanthe* helped, because both produce, in toxic doses, trismus, tetanus and convulsions, with a red face, and opisthotonus. However, this child did not arch the head and spine backwards, but flexed forward, and went pale during each fit.

The case demonstrates that homeopathic medication can be added to conventional medication. The child continued taking sodium valproate though he discontinued taking nitrazepam. In this case a higher potency (30c) of *Artemisia* appeared more effective than a low potency (3c).

Artemisia vulgaris (which contains the alkaloid artemisinin) was a popular drug known to the Greeks and Romans, and in later times was much used for treating epilepsy and spasms of children (presumably in material doses). Hering recommends it for irregular or deficient menstruation associated with epileptic convulsions. Boericke (*Pocket Manual of Homoeopathic Materia Medica*) advises it for childhood epilepsy, especially for girls reaching puberty, and Clarke (*Dictionary of Practical Materia Medica*) for 'epilepsy from menstrual disturbances'.

I rarely prescribe *Artemisia*, but have two adult female patients whose epilepsy is not strictly controlled by sodium valproate and whose fits increase if their period is overdue. By taking *Artemisia* during the premenstrual week it would appear that the frequency of their fits has been reduced.

MENIÈRE'S DISEASE TREATED WITH *CHENOPODIUM*

CASE 7

A 54-year-old manufacturing jeweller developed tinnitus and increasing deafness in his left ear 'due to the hammering in the factory'. He was already 90% deaf in his right ear following a mastoid operation in 1962, as a consequence of which he had attended the Ear and Throat Hospital regularly at six-month intervals for the last twenty-five years. He could not tolerate using a hearing aid in his left ear, because it only increased his tinnitus, but without an aid he could not understand conversation – 'words were just a jumbled noise'. Two years earlier he was supplied with a hearing aid for his right ear, with which he could now hear conversation. Three years ago the tinnitus in the left ear diminished, and the deafness increased. At the same time he started getting attacks of vertigo and vomiting, which the hospital diagnosed as Menière's disease. Initially the attacks occurred at about eight week intervals, lasting usually between one to three hours, but sometimes as long as nine hours.

Treatment with conventional drugs had failed, apart from cinnarizine, which 'helped a little', and recently the attacks had been getting more frequent, coming every two weeks and becoming more severe. He stated that the uncertainty, severity and frequency of the attacks was beginning to unnerve him and make him feel insecure. He no longer felt safe, or confident, to drive any distance. At his last visit to his GP he apparently had been told that conventional medicine had nothing further to offer him; hence his request for homeopathic treatment.

On 8.10.85, at his first consultation, he presented as a cheerful, normotensive man (BP 140/80). He had never smoked, did not drink alcohol, avoided drinking coffee, and only drank tea in moderation. He was overweight at 92kg (203lb), height 1.75m (5ft 9in). Apart from his aural pathology, physical examination was otherwise unremarkable. He was free from nasal catarrh, and in fact only recalled two occasions in the last ten years when he had suffered from catarrh.

His most significant symptoms from a homeopathic aspect were:

Deaf, yet intolerance of loud noise.
'Loud noise hurts me', e.g. singing in church.
'The noise of traffic gets on my nerves. It is unbearable, it sets my deaf ear pulsating and ringing, and makes me miserable.'

'Deaf to thunder.' Dependent on hearing aid.

He observed: 'It is strange to be deaf and yet sensitive to noise.'

By stroking the skin in front of his left ear he produced numbness of the skin on the left side of his face, and tinnitus 'like the sound of a violin string being plucked'.

Treatment

Chenopodium (Jerusalem oak) 3c three times a day.

Cocculus (Indian cockle) 6c half-hourly in attacks of Menière's.

Cinnarizine 15 mg three times a day.

Stop added salt and sugar.

Start high fibre diet (to help to control his obesity).

12.2.86. No attacks since. Hearing deteriorating in left ear. Weight loss of 3.2 kg (7 lb). Not needed to try *Cocculus*.

Treatment

Chenopodium 30c twice a day at 7-day intervals.

Chenopodium 3c twice a day on the intervening days.

11.6.86. No attacks in the last eight months. Hospital provided a new hearing aid four months ago. Feeling in an 'contented state of mind'. 'I have regained my confidence in driving and going out. I am not living in fear of an attack. I could drive to Scotland now.'

Treatment

Stop cinnarizine.

Chenopodium 30c in the morning at 7-day intervals.

Chenopodium 3c daily on the intervening days.

After two weeks reduce *Chenopodium* 30c to 14-day intervals.

After four weeks try reducing *Chenopodium* 3c to alternate mornings.

15.10.86. No attacks in the last year. Still very sensitive to noise. Replace *Chenopodium* with *Chininum sulphuricum* 3c three times a day until reaction (i.e. symptoms better or worse).

7.1.87. Menière's 200% better. No attacks to date. Feels old self again.

Stopped *Chininum sulph.* and reverted to *Chenopodium*, as tinnitus had returned. No change in the hypersensitivity to noise since discontinuing *Chininum sulph.*

Treatment

Trial of *Theridion* (orange spider) 30c x 12 doses alternate mornings (to reduce hypersensitivity to noise).

12.4.87 Feeling very well. No attacks since first consultation 18 months ago, when started taking *Chenopodium*. *Theridion* 30c had been ineffective in reducing his hypersensitivity to noise, rather it aggravated it. All therapy was stopped.

9.5.87. 'Perfect.' No further attacks.

Discussion

One of the problems in analysing such a case, where multiple prescriptions have been used, is that it is not possible to be sure which medicine has been effective. In this particular case *Theridion* caused an aggravation to his noise sensitivity, and so may ultimately have been the effective medicine in curing the attack, although one can never be sure. Classical single remedy prescribing is of course preferable, although the overriding factor is the cure of the patient.

As recently as my early years in medicine, oil of chenopodium was the treatment of choice for hookworm and roundworm infestation. It was recognised that it did not kill the worms, but only paralysed them, so they then had to be expelled with a purgative. The drug worked best when given as a mixture of one volume of oil of chenopodium with two volumes of carbon tetrachloride. In treating children the oil was usually given on sugar, one drop per year of age twice or three times a day for two days, followed by a purge.

However, there were serious problems because:

- The active component of chenopodium is ascaridole, which 'is deadly to man and worm'; the respective lethal doses lie near one another, and its reported percentage in the oil has varied from 33% to 98%.
- The size of drops varied with different droppers, and there was catastrophic confusion between 45 drops of the International Dropper (2.2ml) and 45 minims (3ml). Numerous deaths have followed the latter.
- Even with therapeutic doses, minor toxic effects such as dizziness, nausea, tinnitus and temporary deafness frequently occur.

Kent, in his *Repertory*, lists 90 medicines for treating sensitivity to noise. The sixteen in large black type are: ACON., ASAR., BELL., BOR., CHIN., CHIN. ARS., COFFEA, CONIUM, KALI CARB., NIT. ACID, NUX VOM., OP., SEPIA, SIL., THERID., ZINC.

Surprisingly he does not include *Chenopodium anthelminticum*. In the section on 'Hearing' it is only listed once, and that is under 'Hearing impaired – the human voice'. Even then it is only in italics, whereas PHOS. and SULPHUR are in heavy black type.

Clarke calls *Chenopodium* 'worm-seed' and describes its symptoms as 'Roaring in ears as of cannons going off; deafness. Progressive deafness to human voice, extreme sensitiveness to other sounds (cerebral deafness?) – Tinnitus synchronous with heartbeats.' This precisely describes the patient's symptoms. Clarke lists vertigo as an indication for *Chenopodium*, but does not mention Menière's disease.

Boericke gives, as indications for the use of *Chenopodium*: 'Sudden vertigo, Menière's disease, torpor of auditory nerve. Comparative deafness to sound of voice, but great sensitiveness to sound, as of passing vehicles, aural vertigo.' This again is an accurate description of the patient's condition.

The deafness of *Chenopodium* is not to be confused with that of *Graphites*, which is unique, being the only medicine listed for hearing that improves in noise! 'Hearing impaired – noise ameliorates', GRAPHITES (heavy black type).

Chenopodium has an unusual symptom: 'Intense pain between angle of right shoulder blade near spine through to heart'. *Chelidonium* (celandine) produces a similar pain – slightly more lateral, described as a 'constant pain under the inferior angle of the right scapula'. *Chelidonium* also produces vertigo and is listed far more frequently in Kent, under that heading, than is *Chenopodium*. I personally cannot recall ever using *Chelidonium* for treating vertigo.

Lilienthal defines Menière's disease as 'vertigo of auditory nerve', but only gives details of *Chininum sulph.*, *Cicuta*, *Conium*, *Kalmia lat.* and *Salicylic acid*. Presumably *Chenopodium* had not been proved in 1879, when he edited his second edition. I have only had success with the first and last of these as far as I can remember. In treating Menière's disease I find that Boericke is the most helpful repertory, and gives the widest choice of medicines under 'Vertigo, of labyrinthic origin (Menière's disease)'. He lists, in italics, (i.e. as the most important medicines) *Chenopodium*, *Chininum sulph.*, *Natrum salicylicum*, *Salicylic acid* and *Theridion*. Kent does not include either Menière's or 'aural vertigo'.

There is still one medicine that could be indicated, especially if his condition relapsed and *Chenopodium* failed to control the attacks: *Proteus* is the bowel nosode for conditions associated with cramps and spasms, Menière's and Raynaud's disease. It should also be considered in treating intractable cases of angioneurotic oedema and urticaria, both conditions often being associated with 'prolonged strain'.

MENIÈRE'S DISEASE – TINNITUS TREATED WITH *SALICYLIC ACID*

CASE 8

In 1970, the matron of a nearby hospital had such repeated and severe attacks of Menière's disease that she had to stop work and also ran the risk of losing her driving licence. She had had occasional mild attacks for four years, but had found that conventional drugs controlled these. Her attacks had become more disabling, lasting three to four hours and occurring every two to three days. She was exhausted as a consequence of them. The attacks consisted of giddiness and vomiting with left-sided tinnitus. She also had increasing deafness in the left ear. The giddiness increased the deafness, which recovered when the giddiness subsided. The ENT specialist noted the strange feature that the tinnitus disappeared when she had the giddiness, only to return afterwards. He did exhaustive investigations (mentioning the possibility of surgery as a last resort in this case), and prescribed various vasodilators – nicotinic acid in increasing doses in the first place. She discontinued these as the giddiness became worse and she felt too hot, and the stools became too relaxed.

At this stage I gave her *Natrum salicylicum* 3c four times a day, until reaction. She took three doses that day, and one dose the next morning, and then discontinued the medication as she felt so much better and the giddiness had disappeared. She was so dramatically improved that she asked to be allowed to return to duty, having been off work for the last month on account of her complaint. That was in September 1970, and over the next six months she had two further doses of *Nat. sal.* 10M and remained virtually symptom-free. The consultant was very pleased with her recovery, and I have no doubt attributed it to the vasodilators she was taking (but which had had to be changed twice as the first two kinds upset her).

DIABETIC PERIPHERAL NEUROPATHY

CASE 9

Mrs M.G., age 44, first consulted me on 20.8.82 and gave the following history. She had suffered from diabetes since six years old and had had insulin twice daily for the last thirty-seven years, including thirty-two years on protamine zinc insulin. All this time she had been under regular hospital surveillance, and was currently maintained on pork isophane insulin 40 strength, 9 units twice daily. Her diabetes was still unstable, she could not control her glycosuria satisfactorily, and still had severe attacks of hypoglycaemia.

Ten years ago she had developed severe diabetic peripheral neuropathy and in recent years had had a frozen shoulder (left), a transposition of her left ulnar nerve (1981), and an operation for a left median carpal tunnel syndrome (1981). To add to her problems she suffered from angina pectoris and fluid retention.

For the previous year her medication had included high doses of non-steroidal anti-inflammatory drugs, high doses of analgesics and diuretics. Despite this heavy dosage with analgesics she was still in considerable pain. She complained of:

1) Severe pain 'like someone permanently sticking needles in the soles of my feet' and 'like electric shocks in my legs and bottom', especially severe at night, and on waking. The pain was better for cold, so that she spent most evenings sitting on a rubber ring with her legs exposed.

2) Severe cramping pains on sitting, necessitating constant changing of position; she had to stop the car three times during the twenty-mile journey to her consultation, and be helped out, to stretch her legs, to ease her pain. These pains began about ten years previously, but had been very much worse for the last year.

3) Loss of sensation in her legs, and loss of balance after sitting so that she had 'to be helped to get balanced on attempting to stand up and walk'. She was only able to walk about twenty yards.

4) Total bilateral anaesthesia of lower limbs, up to her thighs. (She demonstrated how she could insert a hypodermic needle full length into different parts of her thigh without any feeling of pain.)

5) Inability to dorsiflex her ankles, so that on the days when she was still able to drive, she had to lift the whole of her foot off the pedal.

6) Inability to stand unless wearing shoes with adequate high heels.

7) Paraesthesia of upper limbs. 'My arms go numb, so I don't know where they are. It makes me drop my knitting.' Wrists and fingers stiff and numb on waking, with 'jumping pains' better for movement.

8) Dependency on others, needing help to get up in the morning and dress. 'I have to come down stairs on my bottom. All joints from the waist down are painful and stiff on waking, easing with movement.'

9) Profound lassitude.

10) Ulcers of her ankles and feet, and recurrent sepsis around her toe-nails. The ulcers started about five years ago, invariably following minor trauma, lasted six to eight weeks, and there was usually at least one present at a time.
11) Fluid retention. 'If I don't take my diuretics I rapidly gain two stone (12.7 kg/28 lb) in weight.'

Treatment

As her most pressing need was for relief of pain, I prescribed mainly on her particular symptoms:

Phytolacca 3c (pokeroot) three times a day until improvement.
If no response after ten days change to *Agaricus* 3c (fly agaric mushroom) four times a day.

I instructed her to continue taking all her conventional medication, explaining that in her case homeopathic medication was an additional therapy, but that she could reduce the analgesics if she found the pain diminishing.

Phytolacca in its provings produces:

- Shooting pains like electric shocks, that radiate, especially in the distribution of the brachial plexus, and sciatic distribution.
- Rheumatic type of pains – very like those produced by *Rhus tox.*, i.e. worse in the mornings, worse wet, cold and at night.
- Better for warmth and dry but worse for motion (like *Bryonia*).

Agaricus (which contains muscarin) in contrast produces:

- Jerkings, twitchings, tremblings, chorea-like movements, and itching.
- Neuralgia – painful spasms, tearing pains, with numbness, coldness and tingling, worse cold, better for movement.
- Paralysis of lower limbs.
- Pains as if pierced by needles of ice.
- Itching of toes, and feet, as if frozen – burning, itching, redness.
- Swelling as if from frostbite (hence its use homeopathically in the treatment of chilblains).
- Ataxia.

At her second visit two months later (22.10.82) she reported that she was sleeping better. She had discontinued the conventional anti-inflammatory drugs, and reduced her analgesics from eight to two daily. 'I have only taken four in the last four days.'

She considered *Agaricus* helped more than *Phytolacca*, and after three weeks had reduced the dose to *Agaricus* 3c one at night only. 'It stops me waking up.'

She could now sit for short spells without her cushion.

Treatment

Zincum metallicum 200c x 1, repeating every fourteen days if required. Try withholding *Agaricus*.

22.12.82. '*Zincum* helped for three to four days, but the best improvement came after reverting to *Agaricus*.'

'Occasionally wakened by restless legs, then I have to walk the room.'

Treatment

Zincum met. 10M x 1 and try *Zincum met.* 6c three times a day in place of *Agaricus*.

19.1.83. '*Zincum* 6c suits better than *Agaricus* 3c.'

She complained of burning, swollen, hot, stinging wrists, swollen feet and 3.2 kg (7 lb) weight gain each evening (despite diuretics), which disappeared each morning.

Treatment

Apis 3c four times a day until relief.

2.3.83. Discontinued all conventional analgesics for last three weeks. *Apis* relieved both wrist pains and fluid retention dramatically.

'I can now move more easily, and walk fifty yards, the best for over a year. I have no jumping pains, and the numbness is considerably improved.'

9.5.83. No analgesics for the last three months.

Sleeping more comfortably – less dependent, more mobile. Takes *Zincum* 6c one to two doses on days when pain returns, on average on four days each fortnight.

She stated that one or two doses of *Zincum* 6c predictably stopped her pain. However, she complained of persistent dyspepsia for the last month with hunger pains, eased by cimetidine and metoclopramide.

She was awaiting a cholecystogram.

She was intolerant of fats, admitted to being very emotional; she liked change. ('My husband is often surprised when he comes home because I've had the furniture rearranged.')

Treatment

Pulsatilla 30c (wind flower) four times a day until reaction.

14.5.83. Her dyspepsia was already much improved, 'better than in all the previous month'.

12.9.83. The neuralgia is still controlled adequately with *Zincum met.* 6c. 'The pain goes within one hour of taking a tablet.' Her cholecystogram and gastric investigations were all unremarkable.

11.10.83. Not taken any conventional analgesics for the last eight months.

Pulsatilla no longer eased her dyspepsia, but surprisingly she found that *Zincum met.* 6c did, and that it was more effective than metoclopramide. She needed to take it four times a day, otherwise her gastralgia lasted for hours. Her neuralgic pains were still controlled effectively with *Zincum*. She could now walk three quarters of a mile – a big improvement on her original limit of twenty yards.

Discussion

McLeod (*Medicine* 1980; 34:1756) states that 'the most common form of peripheral neuropathy in diabetes mellitus is a symmetrical, predominantly sensory, polyneuropathy. When there is severe sensory impairment, perforating ulcers of the feet and neuropathic joints may occur, with associated sensory ataxia (diabetic pseudotabes). Motor and sensory conduction are impaired. Isolated peripheral nerve lesions are common, particularly carpal tunnel syndrome, ulnar nerve lesions at the elbow and radial, femoral and lateral popliteal nerve palsies.'

The same author lists the metals and industrial agents that cause peripheral neuropathy, and includes arsenic, lead, mercury, thallium and gold (but not zinc).

The reason I considered *Zincum met.* might be even more effective than *Agaricus* was because of two previous occasions when I had prescribed it for diabetic patients with peripheral neuropathy. Both had received protamine zinc insulin (PZI) for many years, and both found that low potency *Zincum met.* afforded considerable relief. This patient had had PZI for thirty-two years, and displayed several of the features one associates with the provings of *Zincum*.

Severe pain, twitching and trembling of her lower limbs with marked weakness.

Pain temporarily relieved by motion, making her constantly move her legs and change position ('restless legs', 'fidgety feet').

Very sensitive soles of her feet.

Profound prostration, 'feeling totally exhausted', with mental apathy.

Dyspepsia.

She claims that *Zincum* affords more relief than *Agaricus*, which certainly helped her.

Summary

This case is presented for teaching purposes, not to attempt to prove that *Zincum met.* in potency will predictably alleviate, or improve diabetic neuropathy, but to illustrate the use of homeopathy in apparently intractable cases of nerve damage. It is interesting to speculate on the possible association between her prolonged use of PZI and the apparent benefit she obtains from low potency *Zincum met.*

It is also worth observing that it often happens, as in this case, that more than one remedy in low potency may help a patient, though none may be the exact simillimum; obviously the one whose clinical picture most nearly matches the total cluster of the patient's symptoms should prove the most effective. Finally, this patient found more benefit from low potency *Zincum* than high – confirming common experience that where there is advanced pathological change, with physical rather than mental symptoms, low potency prescribing is generally the most successful.

NEURALGIA

CASE 10

A 63-year-old man attended because of severe intractable post-herpetic neuralgia, which resulted from an attack of facial shingles ten years previously.

A few weeks later he had had a stroke. To protect the eye on the affected side of his face, an ophthalmic surgeon had sutured the eyelids together, as a temporary measure.

The supraorbital area on the affected side was extremely hyper-sensitive, so that the least touch produced an intensely sharp pain 'like hot needles'. Paradoxically, he could tolerate (and get some relief from) firm pressure. By day he was pain-free, as long as nothing touched the tender part; by night he was wakened constantly by a hot throbbing pain, which was slightly eased by cold applications. Carbamazepine was the only medication that had mitigated the pain, but it 'doped' him so much that he discontinued taking it.

He had attended a pain clinic for two years, and the only effective treatment had been acupuncture, which helped initially, but the benefit wore off.

I prescribed, in order:

Mezereum 6c (spurge olive) (see Boericke, 'Head' and 'Eyes'),
Arsenicum alb. 30c,
Verbascum 6c (mullein), none of which made the slightest difference.

Finally I prescribed *Magnesia phosphorica* 30c twice a day as required. He was delighted with this medicine, finding that one tablet eased the pain at night, and controlled the hypersensitivity by day for six to eight hours. Six months later he reported that he had never felt so well in the last ten years, and the *Mag. phos.* was still effective, though he was using it less frequently.

I had deferred giving *Mag. phos.* originally because it is indicated for pains aggravated by cold and relieved by warmth – the reverse of his symptoms. However, the character of the pain was typical, and the unusual modality of worse for touch and better for pressure was more significant. This 'strange, rare and peculiar' modality is listed in Kent's repertory in the section 'Face', where three rubrics are relevant in this case:

'Pain, pressure ameliorates', *Mag. phos.* is the only medicine in bold black type.

'Pain, touch aggravates' – includes *Mag. phos.*

'Pain, warmth ameliorates' – only *Ars. alb.*, *Hepar sulph.*, *Mag. phos.* and *Silica* are in bold black type.

The action of *Mag. phos.* in this case is not likely to be psycho-somatic, inasmuch as the patient had already tried three previous medicines, all identical in colour, shape, size and taste, and could well have become disillusioned with homeopathy, before taking this fourth, and apparently effective remedy.

Mag. phos. is usually more effective than *Colocynth* in treating abdominal colic and dysmenorrhoea, if the patient gets more relief from applied heat to the abdomen than from pressure.

PARAPARESIS

CASE 11
This was a small, thin, very active woman who, at fifty years of age, still regularly cycled six miles to work as a cleaner. In January 1970 she developed a typical endogenous depression and was referred

to a local psychiatric hospital where she had a course of out-patient electroconvulsive therapy, which failed to relieve her. She then developed persistent diarrhoea, which did not respond to diazepam and sulphasalazine in full doses. This lasted six months, despite various alterations in her hospital treatment. Her depression deepened, so she was admitted to a psychiatric hospital, but on further investigation she was found to have difficulty in walking and a mild hemiparesis. She was transferred to another psychiatric hospital, with a medical unit, and where the physician had a special interest in neurology. She was exhaustively investigated, but no cause for her symptoms found.

I was attached to this hospital as a clinical assistant, and was able to observe the woman's downhill progress at close quarters.

By now, the patient was totally dependent and a picture of abject misery. She was no longer able to stand unsupported, or get up unaided out of a chair. She could not balance, she could not dress herself, and could scarcely feed herself. She had to have a nurse to help her to walk to the toilet; and her mental dejection increased at the same rate as her physical helplessness. At this stage her relatives insisted on taking her out of hospital, as nothing more appeared to be being done for her. The hospital acquiesced, on the understanding that she would be admitted to the neurological unit of another hospital when a bed was available. Accordingly, she was brought home after three months in hospital, and I visited her on 25.9.70.

The picture, then, was of this debilitated, depressed, underweight woman, complaining of giddiness and urinary frequency and in-continence, who had a cold feeling from the waist down to the groins, and weakness and trembling of the left arm and leg. She felt cold, and liked a blazing fire, and at night felt 'as if she were lying in a wet bed'. Her neck muscles were so weak that she could not easily hold her head up, and she was irritable and prostrated. She 'trembled inwardly', and when she fell down, could not get up without assistance. In brief she was completely dependent and housebound.

On 13.10.70 I gave her one dose of *Cocculus* 10M and a placebo three times a day to follow, and three days later she walked, with help, the half mile from her own house to her mother's house. She began cooking her husband's meals.

By 20.10.70 she was able to walk unaided without her walking-frame, using only a walking stick. She still had her weakness and trembling of her left limbs, and a left extensor plantar response. I ordered her some more placebo. A week later her condition was relapsing, and she had a second dose of *Cocculus* 10M. That week she went shopping.

On 3.11.70 she was walking the half mile to her mother's house unaided, and was doing her washing and housework without help. She was still very weak, very slow and very tremulous, and dispirited, as she had always been such an active woman before her illness.

At this stage I bumped into the consultant physician who had treated her in hospital, and who was still of the opinion that she had some intra-cranial vascular or neoplastic pathology. He could not understand how she could have improved, and turned to his registrar and said, 'But we didn't give her anything, did we?' At that time I did not enlighten him as to the homeopathic treatment, because I thought I would wait and watch a little longer. If I had said it was picrotoxin, which is the alkaloid of *Cocculus*, I don't suppose he would have minded, unless I had added, 'in an ultramolecular potentised form!'

She was admitted to another neurological unit in early December; and again all her blood, biochemical, CSF, EEG, and X-ray investigations were normal, including brain scan and carotid angiogram. On examination they found she still had left facial weak-ness, a coarse tremor of the left arm, and quite marked bradykinesia (slowing of movement) of the left side of the body. Her gait was cautious but not ataxic. They diagnosed her as having arteriosclerotic Parkinsonism, and postulated that this might have followed a stroke. They started her on L-dopa, and she continued on this therapy in increasing doses.

She had further doses of *Cocculus* 10M on 2.12.70 and 22.12.70, and on 20.1.71 and 2.3.71, and continued to improve very slowly.

Discussion

Many of the features of this patient's illness are represented in the materia medica of *Cocculus* (the Indian cockle). These are:-

- Profound sadness
- Vertigo
- Paralysis of facial nerve
- Lameness and trembling in limbs. Numb and unsteady.
- One-sided paralysis

It is in bold type in Kent in the general rubric of 'trembling', and in italics in 'trembling of the hand', and in bold type in 'trembling of the hand during eating', a symptom found in Parkinson's disease.

MULTIPLE SCLEROSIS

CASE 12

Her multiple sclerosis started when she was thirty-six years old, nine years previously, and had progressed to the stage where she had difficulty in walking from the car park in the city centre to the nearby office where she worked. She had been under a neurologist all that time, until a month earlier when she decided that she was not going to continue taking conventional medication, as it was not helping her. She repeatedly had 'shooting pains' up her legs, which felt very weak. Her extremities were always cold, and her legs trembled and twitched at night in bed.

I prescribed *Menyanthes* (buckbean) 6c three times a day, which seemed appropriate but 'it made no difference'.

I then tried *Lathyrus* (chickpea) 6c three times a day, which did not help either, but it is indicated for painless paralysis of the legs, with exaggerated reflexes. In her case she definitely suffered from pain.

Finally I gave her *Thallium* 3c three times a day, and she noticed an immediate response. 'The pain is less, my legs feel stronger, and I can walk further. I feel reassured when I take the tablets.'

She experimented with the dosage, and found the optimum regime was a five-day course, followed by a three-day interval. She continued this with benefit for the next three and a half years until she left the district and I lost touch with her.

Thallium toxicity results in progressive paralysis of the lower limbs with 'most horrible neuralgic spasmodic shooting pains, like electric shocks'. There is an associated cyanosis of the extremities, and trembling. Hence the homeopathicity of *Thallium* in her case.

TRANSVERSE MYELITIS

CASE 13

A 34-year-old woman had been diagnosed as having transverse myelitis fourteen years previously, and decided to seek homeopathic treatment as her condition was deteriorating. Her legs were becoming weaker so that she could not stand for long, and her backache increased. She also began to twitch in her legs: 'It isn't a jerk, but just a disturbing twitching sensation that even wakes me in the night.'

I prescribed *Picric acid* 6c three times a day.

A month later she felt stronger and her backache was slightly eased. She said all the twitching had gone. When asked how quickly the tablets had worked she replied, 'I just took them on a regular basis and didn't get the twitching any longer. My teatime dose stops my night attacks. I had had the twitchings continuously for four months.'

Picric acid and *Phosphoric acid* are frequently indicated in treating the post-viral syndrome and myalgic encephalomyelitis (ME), where there is prostration with mental and physical exhaustion. The modalities of the two medicines differ: *Picric acid* is indicated where the physical symptoms predominate, and is worse for sleep, warmth and hot weather and the wet; the headache is occipital and often (like *Silica*) relieved by tight bandaging. In contrast, *Phosphoric acid* is indicated where the apathy, confusion and loss of memory predominate, with a crushing headache involving the vertex, and often associated with vertigo.

EPILEPSY

CASE 14

This is the case of Matthew, who was six years old at the time of his first consultation. When three years old he had a viral infection, followed by a complete left hemiplegia, from which he slowly recovered. He had a residual flexure contracture of his left hand, but could extend his left elbow. At that time his parents were living in the Midlands, so he was admitted to a Midlands hospital, and was under a local paediatrician until the family moved to Wales, to take over a post office.

At the beginning of October 1985 Matthew started having atypical fits; both his arms would deviate to the left, he would gently go down on one knee, fall on to his face, and be unable to get up again. His eyes remained open, he appeared to be conscious and aware of what was happening, yet was unable to answer. He salivated profusely. As a result of these episodes he had become slightly ataxic, was frightened to climb or descend stairs in case he fell, and so started coming downstairs on his knees. He had hurt himself many times through falling. The attacks only lasted a few seconds.

On 11.11.85 Matthew's father telephoned me for an urgent appointment for him, and to ask for advice as to any appropriate homeopathic treatment for him to be going on with until I could see him, as he had had five or six fits every day without respite for the last six weeks. The father knew a little about homeopathy, and Matthew was regularly given *Arnica* after each fall. I suggested he gave him *Nux vomica* 30c twice daily as a first aid remedy until I could see him. *Nux vomica* contains strychnine and therefore has spasm and convulsions in its materia medica. Significantly, the eyes also remain open (as in this boy's case).

A week later, on 18.11.85, the parents brought him and were delighted to report he had not had a single fit since his first dose of *Nux vomica* 30c. More than that, Matthew was not losing his balance, as previously. He was brighter, and more alert, and not complaining of tiredness at the end of each school week. He was now able to walk to school much better, not needing to be held all the time. His teacher had noted a 'remarkable improvement'.

He appeared to be a quiet, outgoing lad who had cold clammy feet, loved savoury food, and was relatively thirstless. His mother remarked, 'I have to push him to drink.' She also stated that Matthew could be very defiant at times, and had temper tantrums.

I continued the *Nux vomica* but in a 200c potency from time to time, and also prescribed *Calcarea phosphorica* 200c as his 'constitutional medicine', to be taken at intervals of approximately three weeks. I emphasised to the parents that they should take any conventional medication prescribed, since homeopathic treatment, in Matthew's case, would be additional to conventional medication.

About two weeks later I received a photocopy of a letter from a Herefordshire paediatrician to Matthew's previous paediatrician in the Midlands. 'Thank you for your letter about Matthew. I saw him for an initial review today. As you say, he has had many fairly stereotyped attacks where the left arm shoots out and he falls down onto his right knee. He says that his mouth feels full of saliva. On occasions he has fallen right down and has had difficulty getting up. There is no change in consciousness, incontinence or post-ictal sleep. These episodes last only a few seconds. He has recently been seen by a homeopathic doctor and has gone three weeks without further attacks. This is certainly unusual for him.

On examination he is very well, but he has the obvious mild left hemiplegia.

I would have thought that these attacks were epileptic, or possibly extrapyramidal involuntary movements. I will arrange for a further EEG. If the attacks recur he will need anticonvulsants. Carbamazepine would be the obvious drug of first choice, and I would be very tempted to try him with a small dose initially.'

On 20.2.86 I received a copy of a report on Matthew, this time to his general practitioner:

Matthew, who is now six, developed an encephalopathy at the age of three and was left with a left-sided hemiparesis and persistent fitting, which involved the left side of his body up until 18 November last year, when he was started on homeopathic medicine. Since then he has had no further fitting and is doing well at school and copes very well with his moderate left hemiparesis.

It was unusual to find that the EEG which was performed at Christmas showed abnormality of the left hemisphere, not the right, as would be expected. We will not investigate Matthew further unless he has any more fits and would like to see him in six months time in the clinic.

On 27.2.86 Matthew attended his second consultation. He had had a 'small fit' during the car journey home from his first appointment three months previously. He was often 'travel sick'. He was then given another dose of *Nux vomica* 200c, and had not had a fit since. He was progressing very well at school, walked better, but always kept his left arm behind his back, with his wrist flexed – like the position of the arm when receiving a 'policeman's tip'. He now had chilblains and cold hands and feet.

Treatment

Agaricus 200c x 1.
Agaricus 3c four times a day until his chilblains disappeared.
Homeopathic travel tablets. (These contain *Apomorphine*, *Cocculus*, *Nux vomica*, *Petroleum*, *Staphysagria*, *Tabacum* and *Theridion*.)

On 1.5.86 his parents reported that Matthew had had a relapse; he was very tired by the end of the spring term, and during the Easter holidays had been having five or six minor fits each day. They only lasted a few seconds, and he did not go down on his knee. 'His eyes could follow you, though he could not speak. *Nux vomica* had not made any difference.' As a substitute I decided to try *Strychninum*, the active principle of *Nux*.

Treatment

Strychninum 12c twice daily.

After a week's treatment with *Strychninum* the pattern of the fits changed, and decreased to two morning fits only. The parents then independently switched the medication back to *Nux vomica* 200c twice daily for three days, and the fits ceased altogether.

On 29.8.86 he again attended. He had had no fits since May, but was embarrassed by his left arm that 'floated' uncontrollably in an athetoid manner. He had again become exhausted by the end of the summer term.

Treatment

Scutellaria 3c (skullcap) three times a day.

Scutellaria did not appreciably control his left arm movements, though these have decreased with time, but appeared to improve his lassitude and apathy.

A year later, on 8.9.87, the parents reported Matthew had his first relapse of fits since May 1986. The fits, however, were mild, and only occurred two or three times a day. They associated this relapse with his becoming very tired, again at the end of the long summer term. 'His left arm sticks out, and he grins, as if to say "It's happening again". He is doing well at the local school, is above average in his reading, and average in maths.' He only sees the consultant annually and is not on any conventional medication. The parents feel they can cope perfectly well with him, and he is no longer a trial to them.

On 23.9.87 Matthew woke up with a total left hemiparesis from which he was fully recovered within half an hour. He had a second similar episode an hour later. Following this, his left hand started going into flexure spasms, as often as ten times a day. *Cuprum met.* 3c four times a day was given, and the incidence of these spasms fell to two to three times a day during the next forty-eight hours, and ceased altogether after a week. He still gets his turns, when his arm 'floats', and he salivates, but these episodes only occur two or three times a day, and only last a few seconds. He remains conscious throughout.

Discussion

If *Nux*, which contains strychnine, or *Strychninum* had failed to control Matthew's minor 'turns', there were still other homeopathic anticonvulsants to be considered. As the precipitating factor in both relapses appeared to be physical and nervous exhaustion, *Scutellaria* could have been be indicated. This plant, the skullcap, resembles the dead nettle and is a tried and useful medicine for treating 'post-flu' debility. At one time used by North American Indians to ease dysmenorrhoea, the early American homeopaths used it in potency 'for its calming effects on the nervous system', the way their European contemporaries used Valerian. It also produces muscle twitching and spasms. Nowadays it should be considered for treating the 'post-viral syndrome'. Matthew's hemiplegia followed a viral infection.

In summary, Matthew has had no major fits where he has fallen since taking *Nux vomica*, whereas they had occurred consistently five or six times daily for six weeks. He was not yet fully recovered but the parents were delighted; the paediatricians also seemed impressed. I have no further knowledge of his progress since that visit.

SEVERE LEARNING DIFFICULTIES WITH EPILEPSY

CASE 15

In April 1982 Bonita, a 12-year-old epileptic girl, was brought to see me for homeopathic treatment. She had severe learning difficulties and was mute, dribbling, and inaccessible. She could not walk, was incontinent of urine day and night, and totally dependent. She was 1.37 m (4 ft 6 in) tall and weighed 44.5 kg (98 lb). She attended a 'special school', and one of the staff came with her and her mother to the consultation. She was under hospital surveillance and her daily medication was:

- clonazepam 3.5 mg
- clobazam 30 mg
- carbamazepine 700 mg

Despite all this anticonvulsant therapy, she was having, on average, fifty major fits each day. The teacher confirmed the mother's statement that 'she is in and out of fits all the time, more in than out'. She recently had been in status epilepticus, and required paraldehyde. The fits could be induced by excitement and by playing with certain objects. The mother was exhausted, and to exacerbate her problems, she had to change Bonita's nappies three times each night.

I first of all insisted that they must on no account alter the medication that either their GP or the hospital were giving, and gave *Baryta carb.* 10M to be taken at one-monthly intervals. I furthermore gave some *Nux vomica* 200c granules, which they could try placing on the child's lips or tongue during a epileptic attack. Finally I prescribed *Equisetum* 3c (scouring rush, mare's tail), to be taken one at night, to see if this would help reduce the nocturnal urinary incontinence.

Five months later (6.9.82), I saw the girl again; there had been some encouraging improvements:

She was not incontinent, and had been out of nappies for the last three months, the first time in her life.

The number of fits had fallen to one or two per day and were much less severe. Usually only one dose of *Nux vomica* 200c was needed in each fit, and she was better in ten minutes; in a bad attack she would need two to three doses at fifteen-minute intervals before the fit was controlled.

She was not dribbling, as previously.

She could feed herself with help, and could now pull her socks off, though not put them on.

She was 'beginning to make noises, which was quite unusual.'

The mother stated that at the last out-patient attendance, when she told the consultant paediatrician about the additional homeopathic therapy, he had said 'I can't argue against it, the improvement is so obvious.'

A year later the parents' marriage broke up and Bonita had some very severe attacks, finally necessitating hospital admission and a change of medication. Her mother found that *Nux vomica* 200c, given at the onset of a fit, reduced its duration from one and a half hours to half an hour. In all her epileptic attacks she kept her eyes open. The mother was convinced that the domestic stress at that time was responsible for Bonita's relapse. Since the mother's remarriage to a 'caring father', the domestic situation had been very happy and Bonita had been much more settled. Her revised daily medication, which she still took, was:

- sodium valproate 1200 mg
- clonazepam 6 mg

She originally had been given sodium valproate, but had to discontinue it as it made her so nauseated. It also made her hair fall excessively. Now, as she is older, she can tolerate this drug better, and the bouts of nausea are alleviated by *Nux vomica* 200c. The effect on her hair is minimal.

The last report that I had of her was when she was eighteen years old and her mother reported that at that time (September 1987) Bonita could walk for about twenty minutes in the park, if somebody held her hands. She was having four or five petit mals a day, and only an occasional grand mal, if she became upset. She communicated with sign language when she wanted to go to the toilet. She still had occasional lapses of enuresis. On these occasions her mother then started giving *Equisetum* 3c each night, and within a day or two Bonita was dry again.

The mother continued giving *Equisetum* each night for about a month (presumably to be on the safe side), during which time Bonita's enuresis became completely controlled. Then regularly, after this duration of medication with *Equisetum*, she had two consecutive nights of incontinence, which her mother interpreted as an aggravation from *Equisetum*. (I had warned her about the possibility of aggravation following overtreatment.) She then discontinued the *Equisetum*, and Bonita remained continent by night for the next two or three months. I instructed her in future to discontinue the *Equisetum* sooner, after it had controlled the incontinence. She was delighted with her progress, and was giving her *Baryta carb.* 10M at approximately three-month intervals.

RECURRENT REJECTION OF SHUNT

CASE 16

On 22.12.86 I was telephoned by the house surgeon of a neurosurgeon to ask me if I could see, as soon as possible, a child in his unit. The problem was longstanding – the girl was hydrocephalic, had had a meningocele closed on the first day of life, and subsequently had her hydrocephalus treated with a ventriculo-peritoneal shunt at the age of one month. After a long history of repeated admissions for possible blocked shunts, revision was carried out in September 1983, when she was just two years old. The ventricular end of the catheter had been replaced but the wound was constantly becoming infected, and breaking down, so that the shunt had already been replaced nearly thirty times.

She was only five and a half years old and had spent much of her life in hospital. The causal organism that was recovered each time was *Staphylococcus albus*, and despite vigorous intravenous antibiotic therapy the wound usually took a month to heal. She had been readmitted in May 1986, when her shunt again blocked, and been critically ill with septicaemia and bacteraemia; her condition had been 'touch and go'. During this admission she developed epileptiform seizures. She was only discharged at the beginning of December 1986, and three weeks later was again readmitted with her neck wound discharging pus, and the shunt once again 'rejected' – hence the urgency. I visited the child in the ward the next day (23.12.86).

The girl was Indian, hydrocephalic, spastic, unable to walk, and doubly incontinent. She had an intravenous infusion through which vancomycin was being administered, and she was catheterised every three hours. Despite all this she was a happy child who mixed well with the other children and was popular with the nurses. I first had a chat with her father, and then we all went to see her in the ward. She was eating biscuits as we arrived, and apparently was 'always eating', no longer craving for sweets, but asking for crisps and salty foods. Periodically she helped herself to the glass of milk on her locker, and the moment she had finished it she called out, in a demanding voice, 'nurse, more cold milk'. She drank cold milk in preference to water, or pop, and was not on anticonvulsants or other medication that could account for her thirst.

Although her father was with her she treated me with suspicion and reserve, and was obviously very nervous of strangers. She was attention-seeking, calling out unnecessarily to the different nurses who walked past the end of her bed. She would not let me hold her hand.

The homeopathic treatment I proposed was:-

Day 1.   *Tuberculinum* 10M, three doses taken in one day,
Day 2.   *Staphylococcus albus nosode* 30c, one daily. After two
          weeks reduce to one alternate day.
Day 8.   Start *Phosphorus* 30c twice daily, at weekly intervals.

I proposed to review her medication after one month.

The neurosurgeon wrote to me on 26.4.87, saying: 'This child has enjoyed very good health since commencing your medicine, although there is still a tendency for scab formation over the scalp incision. I enclose photocopies of her last discharge summary and my last letters to her GP, and will keep you informed of her subsequent progress.'

The letter to the GP contained the following information: '25.3.87. I have just seen S. whose neck has started to discharge some purulent material again. She is so well in herself, however, that I would really prefer to hold off readmitting her. If months go by and nothing settles I suppose we shall have to consider a new shunt on the other side, but she has had so many problems in hospital that I would prefer to keep her out as long as we can.'

In June of that year 'she was readmitted unnecessarily' for one day at her mother's request, but was discharged the next day as it was found that there was no cause for anxiety. She continued to thrive, was still attending her special school, and was described as 'nice and chubby'.

Discussion

The reasons for prescribing the particular medicines listed were as follows:

Tuberculinum: Her ethnic origin made me suspect that she might have a tuberculous diathesis. She certainly was having regular intermittent fevers, and frequently caught colds. Although generally

68

of a pleasant disposition she did have temper tantrums; and could be stubborn. She craved cold milk and was thirsty, and liked salty foods. She had a voracious appetite, yet was a thin, anaemic-looking child.

Phosphorus: Although showing hostility to me – a stranger – she loved the attention and company of the nurses. She seemed to be a nervous, restless child. She had a feeble constitution, and a liability to catch colds. She was thirsty for cold drinks and had a salt craving.

Staphylococcus albus nosode: This was given empirically because *Staphylococcus albus* was the causal organism on each occasion.

It is interesting to note that in the first five years of life this child rejected her shunt nearly thirty times, and the last occasion before homeopathic treatment necessitated seven months' intensive treatment in hospital. Since having homeopathic therapy she had retained her shunt for the last two years and had picked up in health. She then moved from the district, and the hospital lost touch with her.

MIGRAINE

CASE 17 – Anecdotal but Significant

A few years ago I was taking my family out for the day, and driving through Lichfield at about noon I suddenly developed a very severe left-sided frontal headache, which started at the back of the head and came to settle over the left eye. I attributed it at first to the heat of the day, then to long driving, and then I even blamed the exhaust fumes of the lorry I had been following. I had to stop the car as I was incapacitated by the intensity of the pain.

After a little thought, I decided that although I didn't know the cause, I had a strong suspicion as to the remedy that was indicated. I treated myself to a few granules of *Spigelia* 30c, and in two minutes the headache had entirely lifted and I was able to resume the journey without further return of the headache. The reason *Spigelia*, pink root, worked was that my headache closely simulated the headache produced if one takes an overdose of the tincture of the dried plant.

Indeed, when this American weed was originally proved by volunteers they found a medicine most violent in action and they had to proceed with caution as it produced severe neuralgias, particularly affecting the region of the left eye. The interesting thing in my case was how quickly the remedy acted, because aspirin or other conventional analgesics can only work after they have been absorbed into the blood-stream, which generally takes fifteen to thirty minutes.

CASE 18

A man of 46 presented to me with a twenty-two-year history of migraine. He had attended the Birmingham Eye Hospital without apparent benefit, and his own doctor had tried all the various ergotamine preparations, without relief.

The attacks usually lasted three days, and initially came at least once a month, increasing through the years, first to every fortnight, and prior to consulting me, to as often as every week. The prodromal symptoms were a low occipital pain, which could sometimes be eased by the application of a hot water bottle, and scotoma, which regularly preceded the headache and vomiting by thirty minutes, and which consisted of dazzles in the lower fields of his vision. There was no particular time aggravation, but it was usually a right-sided hemicrania.

The man was lean and sparsely built, with flaxen hair, a light complexion and blue eyes. He had cold, clammy feet and was a chilly person.

I gave him *Silica* 200c, and to his surprise, the attacks rapidly decreased in frequency, duration and severity during the next three months. He started to go for months without a severe attack. He also noticed that his foot sweat was also controlled.

He took an occasional dose of *Silica*, approximately every three months, for the next three years, and then forgot all about it.

His headaches started to return, and he was trying to control them with analgesics when he brought his five-year-old son to me for treatment of his catarrhal deafness. I prescribed *Silica* for him, and then the father remembered his own benefit from *Silica*, and took another dose!

CASE 19

15.10.70. Beryl was a thin, dark haired lady, aged 38 years. She had had migraine for two years, getting worse in the last three months. Now they were lasting twenty-four hours. She had pain in the left supraorbital region (occasionally right), which made her vomit. She was worse for noise, movement, jarring and sitting, and better for dark, pressure, and being alone. I gave her *Bryonia* 30c alternate hours until relief.

6.11.70. She phoned me to say 'Marvellous, the pills worked very quickly.' Requested more.

HEADACHE

CASE 20

A 50-year-old wife of a hospital consultant had suffered from occipital neuralgia for thirty-five years. Her headache had become worse recently, and had occurred on waking every morning for the previous three months. She had had 'neck and back problems' since falling off her horse ten years earlier, which osteopathic treatment had relieved to some extent. However, repeated neck manipulations had failed to cure her headaches.

She described the occipital headache as 'bursting'. It remained localised, did not spread forward, and was not associated with scotomata, nausea or vomiting.

The modalities were: worse on waking, worse at the end of a stressful day.

No association with position, neck pillows, pressure, warmth, cold, movement or jarring.

In the past, she had noticed it was better for walking the dog, and better getting up very early (5 a.m.).

The headache tended to settle during the day.

Being a consultant's wife she had seen many specialists and had many forms of treatment. Her only relief was from strong analgesics.

She had sufficient insight to ask, 'Is it stress related?'

Since I was unable to find a medicine that corresponded to these modalities I enquired into her mental and general symptoms.

She was a sympathetic person who herself craved sympathy, liked being massaged, and cried when upset. She recognised that she was a worrier, with a carcinophobia, and overconcern about her family. She was chilly, bruised easily, was worse in humid weather, thirsty, and preferred salty foods. These and other features pointed to *Phosphorus*.

She was prescribed *Phosphorus* 30c every fourth day.

Five months later she attended again, mainly to report that there had been 'a dramatic response within three days. It was remarkable. I don't know what worked unless it was the tablets. I've not had a severe headache since, despite falling off my bicycle and cricking my neck again two weeks ago.' She had waited this length of time before returning for review to see if the unprecedented remission lasted. After suffering for thirty-five years she had become disillusioned with all the therapies she had tried, and was being cautious. She said her husband was delighted, and when I questioned whether he thought it might all be a psychosomatic response she emphatically denied it.

She also found that *Phosphorus* controlled the aching in her neck and shoulders due to tension when driving.

I instructed her to take *Phosphorus* at longer intervals, i.e. between seven to fourteen days according to response.

This case illustrates the overriding importance of trying to match the patient's mental and general symptoms in exact detail. *Phosphorus*-type headaches usually are:

Worse for heat, motion, lying down, noise, light.

Better for cold, as far as the head is concerned, and eating.

This patient's headache did not have all those classical modalities yet her constitutional medicine undoubtedly was *Phosphorus*, which certainly helped.

Phosphorus is one of the indicated medicines when the patient is suffering from either a bursting congestive headache, or a neuralgic headache, and yet feels hungry and can eat and retain food. I remember one woman who suffered incapacitating morning headaches, and yet regularly breakfasted on buttered toast and coffee. Her headaches responded well to *Phosphorus*.

CASE 21

9.11.71. A 37-year-old lady presented with a six-month history of severe, congestive, premenstrual left frontal headaches, so violent that she had to spend at least one day in bed. The headaches were always worse after sleep and better when the flow was established. They were always left-sided, but sometimes eventually spread slightly across to the right frontal region. They affected her sight, so that she could not see. She was warm-blooded and worse for warmth, worse for noise, and conversation. She was better lying quietly in bed in the dark. She could not tolerate tight clothing round her neck.

Treatment

Lachesis 12c (venom of the bushmaster snake) every four hours until reaction.

31.1.72. Dramatic improvement after the second dose in the last two attacks. 'Far more effective than my strong painkillers (dihydro-codeine)..' Hardly surprising as her features were so typical of *Lachesis*.

CASE 22

24.1.72. A 45-year-old lady was brought by car to the surgery by her husband. She had a very severe right hemicranial headache, which started behind her right eye and spread to the right occiput. She was severely nauseated, and brought a bucket in the car in case she was sick. She had visual disturbances and was worse for movement, even of her eyes, and worse for jarring. She was irritable and uncommunicative, and sat in her chair almost resenting being questioned. She sat holding her head still between both hands, which she pressed tightly to her skull. Her husband answered most of the questions. She was very thirsty during the attacks. I gave her *Bryonia* 30c half-way through interview, and a minute later she volunteered that the pain had nearly gone. Her husband commented 'You look relaxed now.' She was able to walk out of the surgery without experiencing pain on walking.

These modalities are all absolutely typical of *Bryonia*, which indeed worked extremely quickly and well.

CASE 23
20.11.74. Urgent phone request to visit a 24-year-old man with a bursting headache. It had started at 1 a.m. at work in the night, and he was given two co-proxamol tablets by the nurse, which did not help him, so he was sent home. He was very distressed with the headache.

When I visited him, he was lying very still in bed. He was able to move his eyes, but not his head. He had no visual disturbance, nor meningism, and he had not vomited. His pain was better for pressure. He had never suffered from migraine or previous severe headaches.

I gave him a tablet of *Bryonia* 30c and continued talking with him. After a few minutes he began to move his head cautiously, then more vigorously, and wag it in each direction, saying, 'It's gone.' He was so excited that he called his wife up from downstairs, and then was able to get up.

Bryonia is the acute medicine of *Natrum muriaticum*, which if the patient is seen in between attacks, may well be the correct constitutional medicine to use. However, remember never to use *Natrum mur.* in an acute attack, as it may cause a nasty aggravation.

CASE 24
A woman of 33 had a severe headache all afternoon and evening, not relieved by *Nux vomica* and codeine tablets. She was lying in bed feeling very weak, but restless, constantly shifting her position. She could not get warm, despite a hot water bottle, and blankets and an eiderdown round her shoulders – yet she wanted fresh air to her head

and the electric fire turned off. She looked unusually apprehensive and admitted to anxiety, though she did not know the cause. She had nausea and a dry mouth, and wanted sips of water.

She was given *Arsen. alb.* 30c in water, and cold applications to the head, and within half an hour was much improved.

Chapter 6

Allergies

Homeopathy is a wonderful way of treating allergies, because the symptoms produced by the allergic reaction can be matched by the symptoms produced by the homeopathic remedy in crude form. For example, it is a common experience that if you peel onions, and get some of the juice near the face, your eyes will begin to smart and water and your nose will begin to run. Later you will start sneezing and even coughing. You may have a headache, and feel thirsty. These toxic symptoms are in effect a proving of onion juice. Now if a person suffers from hayfever or a head cold that identically simulates the above clinical picture, his condition will improve very quickly if he is given onion juice, but this time in a potentised form, *Allium cepa*. The problem is not just as simple as that, because there are at least two dozen plants or minerals which in toxic doses bring on these symptoms, but each drug picture varies slightly from all the others. It therefore becomes necessary to separate the finer details that distinguish the effects of one plant or mineral poisoning from the others.

The eyebright plant was well known to the ancients and was used by them as an eye medicine. Its bright eyes peep out from the turf of the commons and meadows of the countryside, justifying its botanical name, *Euphrasia*, which means 'to gladden'. Its English name also reminds us of its use. Culpeper says of it: 'If the herb was as much used as it is neglected, it would half spoil the spectacle maker's trade.' *Euphrasia* causes a bland nasal discharge with acrid tears, worse from light and warmth and better in the dark. The cold symptoms are worse at night and lying down, whilst the cough is worse by day and better lying down.

Ambrosia (ragweed) causes hayfever with watering of the eyes and intolerable itching of the eyelids, with a stuffy feeling in the nose and head, and epistaxis.

Sabadilla (cevadilla seeds) causes persistent, violent sneezing, an itchy nose and profuse watery coryza, and may be associated with a left-sided sore throat which is relieved by warm drinks.

The treatment of hayfever illustrates various ways of using homeopathic medicines:

- Immediate relief from local remedies
- Constitutional treatment
- Desensitising treatment

Immediate relief can be afforded by giving the 'like' medicine (that which most closely fits all the symptoms), be it *Allium cepa*, *Euphrasia*, *Sabadilla*, *Ambrosia*, or a number of other remedies.

CASE 25

For example: a patient complained of attacks of rhinitis coming on about once a year, but not at any particular season. She had irritation of the eyes and nose, copious bland discharge from the eyes and nose, and much sneezing.

She was not helped by a decongestant linctus, and I first gave her *Arsenicum iodatum* 12c every two hours, which she stopped taking after three doses because of a severe aggravation. Some days later she returned with new symptoms. There was no sneezing, but profuse lachrymation, coryza and headache. She was worse in the open air, especially if the sunlight was strong. The nasal discharge was acrid.

I changed the remedy to *Allium cepa*, which was again stopped after three doses, this time because the condition had cleared completely. With hindsight, perhaps this change was not necessary, and the *Arsenicum iodatum* achieved the cure, the aggravation having settled.

CASE 26

A man came into a crowded surgery with very pronounced hayfever. His eyes were bloodshot, both his eyes and nose were running, and I had heard him sneezing in the waiting-room. He had had hayfever for many years and had been treated with all the latest antihistamines. He had moved into my district the previous winter, and had delayed coming sooner because he assumed that little could be done.

I had only time to collect a few details, and then gave him one pill of *Euphrasia* 12c. After waiting for five minutes his eyes were neither better nor worse. This meant that the remedy had not touched him, and my hurried diagnosis was incorrect. I asked him a few more questions, and then gave him *Allium cepa*, in the 30c potency because I was more confident in my diagnosis. I asked him to wait outside for ten minutes. Looking through my surgery window, I saw him strolling about in the brilliant sunshine. He had told me that sunshine always made him worse. When I called him in again he was delighted, as he felt much better; his eyes had stopped itching and watering, and moreover they were no longer bloodshot. I gave him a further supply of *Allium cepa* 30c, instructing him on no account to take another pill until his hayfever reappeared, which probably would not be for a few days.

This case illustrates two things:

1) The rapidity of action of a homeopathic remedy in an acute condition – the second pill cleared the conjunctiva of engorged blood vessels in ten minutes. The average antihistamine taken by mouth would not have begun to work in that time.

2) Homeopathy is not a matter of suggestion. Both pills were identical as far as colour, shape, size and taste were concerned. The only difference was that they contained different remedies. The first was ineffective, the second worked dramatically.

The same evening a school mistress came in with bloodshot eyes, suffering from severe hayfever. I gave her *Allium cepa* 30c and recalled her ten minutes later. In that time all her symptoms were relieved, and her eyes had lost their bloodshot appearance.

CASE 27

A lady of thirty-five had a 28-day history of morning coryza after returning from a Swiss holiday. The symptoms consisted of incessant sneezing for two to three minutes, with a clear watery nasal discharge which could soak six handkerchiefs. There were no eye or throat symptoms, and the sneezes would tail off during the morning, to return next day.

A single dose of *Sabadilla* 12c permanently reduced the number of sneezes to one or none, with no accompanying catarrh.

CASE 28

About twenty years ago a consultant was giving himself his third Pollinex injection (a mixture of grass pollens) to desensitise himself against hayfever when, in theatre, he suddenly developed acute bronchospasm and felt faint. He only had time to call out, 'Nurse! Adrenaline!' before he blacked out. He records that when he came round in the coronary care unit he was told that his blood pressure was unrecordable. For the previous three years he had had standard preseasonal courses of injections for hayfever, with no untoward reactions, and no significant benefit. He was advised not to have any more injections, but to try homeopathy.

In his attacks his eyes itched and watered, but were not blood-shot. He had a fluent, clear coryza, but minimal sneezing. His nose felt continually blocked, but cleared temporarily after sneezing. Skin testing did not reveal sensitivity to house dust mite.

On 16th June I prescribed *Sabadilla* 12c alternate hours during his attacks of hayfever, which occurred frequently as the pollen count was rising.

Three days later he phoned to report no improvement. With hind-sight this was understandable. *Sabadilla* works best when the sufferer has bouts of violent sneezing, accompanied by such copious coryza that he could soak half a dozen large handkerchiefs, yet the discharge from the nostrils is so clear that the handkerchiefs could be squeezed out and dried, and remain almost clean.

I suggested he try *Allium cepa* 12c, and if that was ineffective, to switch to *Euphrasia*.

On 7th July he returned from holiday, having found that his eye symptoms had been worse at the seaside, and he had had a severe relapse of his asthma, necessitating full doses of inhaled steroids and bronchodilators. (This was in the days before nebulisers were commonplace.)

As he was most sensitive to timothy grass (*Phleum pratense*) I prescribed it four times a day in 30c potency, with, as a second choice, *Aralia* (American spikenard) 30c.

On 14th July he phoned to express his delight at the great relief of his symptoms that *Phleum* had produced. 'It suits my son as well. I have told various colleagues about it, but their response is to mock me and tell me it's all suggestion. I don't mind, as long as it works. *Aralia* is no use.' Interestingly, *Phleum* was the only medicine out of five that helped him. Since all of them were in tablet form, and indistinguishable in size, shape, colour or taste, his threshold of suggestibility would most likely have been lowered considerably by the time he tried *Phleum*.

Years later I invited him to recount his experience at a symposium on homeopathy at a Birmingham hospital. After explaining the ineffec-tiveness and cost of all the different conventional treatments he had tried in the four years before his near-fatal anaphylactic reaction, he held up his bottle of *Phleum* tablets, and stated how dramatically he had improved since taking them. 'Total cost, 75 pence for 55 tablets.' He then added, 'Each year I take my men in the Territorials to Sweden for training. Because we always go in early summer, the grass pollen count is usually high, and in the past my hayfever has been aggravated by bronchospasm. I have had to stay in the base camp, whilst my men climbed the mountains. Since using *Phleum*, what has stopped me climbing as high as my men is that my legs get tired.'

Later the patient could be *desensitised* against the particular pollen or substance that caused his allergy by giving a homeopathic potency of that substance. Preferably this should be done preseasonally – a month or so before the time at which attacks usually start. Most sufferers usually identify the causal agent, and in those who cannot, skin testing is a quick, safe and simple procedure. Within five minutes a positive response reveals whether the cause is due to mixed pollens, summer flowers, trees, etc., or whether a house dust mite allergy is involved. Specific homeopathic medicines are available to treat all these, and are taken orally. This is called isopathy.

CASE 29

A woman had suffered for thirty years from hayfever which lasted annually from the beginning of April until mid-July.

She was allergic to tree pollens generally, and to silver birch in particular. Antihistamines failed to control the condition and invariably made her drowsy. She stated she had tried everything, and was sceptical about trying homeopathy – she had told her husband my tablets could not possibly help, and she certainly didn't expect them to. She took *Trees* 30c, six doses at the rate of three a day for two days, then one every third day as required. She claimed that she got dramatic relief after eighteen hours, and could not believe it. She had a completely clear season, despite going abroad for a holiday to Poland, where silver birch abounds, and was in blossom.

B3 Trees contains potentised pollen from the ten most allergenic trees in the UK, but does not contain fir or lime.

CASE 30

I lived until recently at a house called The Limes, on account of the nine mature lime trees that flank the drive in close proximity to the house. One summer, the outside of the house was being painted whilst the lime trees were in flower, and one of the painters said he would have to leave the job, as he was too sensitive to the lime pollen. Rather than risk losing a good painter and delaying the work, I suggested he try taking *Lime* 30c daily whilst exposed to the pollen. He agreed, and we were both gratified to discover that he could continue working with minimal discomfort, and without taking any antihistamine preparation.

CASE 31

The same isopathic immunotherapy helped a forester who found he could handle any tree except a Scots pine. By taking a tablet of *Scots pine* 30c each morning on days when he risked exposure, he found he was protected. After a few weeks he was able to reduce the dose to one a week, and eventually to one a month.

CASE 32

I have had two patients who were sensitive to tomatoes. One, a middle-aged man was very fond of his allotment and a keen grower. For the last five years he had been unable to grow tomatoes, or even handle the plants, on account of the irritation and blisters that developed on his skin. He was also sensitive to the sun ever since coming back from the Far East during the war.

    Rhus tox. did not ease his sun dermatitis, but *Antimonium crudum* did. I gave the 12c potency three times a day for four days, and he was most impressed with the way the blisters cleared. It was then he mentioned his tomato sensitivity to me. I gave him *Solanum lycopersicum* (tomato) 30c, one pill twice a day for six doses, and he went all through the summer without any reaction, even though growing tomatoes again. He had a second course the following year, although I am not sure that he really needed it.

CASE 33

The second patient was a short, stout woman, who casually mentioned to me that all her life she had been extremely sensitive to tomato plants. They gave her a streaming cold, and she did not dare even to stand in the doorway of the greenhouse if it contained any tomatoes. I gave her six pills of *Solanum lycopersicum* 30c, one to be taken every morning. Five months later she reported that she had had no relapse; not only had she been able to enter the greenhouse to water the plants, but she had also been able to stay inside to nip off the unwanted side shoots.

CASE 34

A 40-year-old man had suddenly become very allergic to horse dander. As a child he had suffered from asthma and eczema, but thought that he had outgrown his asthma.

    He had recently bought his daughter a pony, but on the three occasions that he had approached it he had had a pronounced reaction, which included lachrymation ('like hayfever'), with swollen itching eyes, fluent coryza, and intense itching of his forehead, followed by a rapid but mild flare-up of eczema. He was loath to have to sell the animal, and asked whether desensitising injections could help him.

I gave him six doses of *Horse dander* 30c, three to be taken at intervals that day, and thereafter one at weekly intervals for the next three weeks.

Neither he nor I anticipated the alarming sequel. Shortly after his last dose, he developed severe bronchospasm, far worse than he had ever previously experienced, and had to be admitted urgently to hospital, where he was given intravenous steroids and antihistamines. At the same time his eczema flared up in an unprecedented way. He had not been in known contact with any animals.

He safely survived the ordeal, and all his respiratory symptoms subsided.

Since then, for the last twenty years, he has been fine. 'I'm absolutely immune now. I can stroke the pony with impunity, and my eyes don't swell or itch, and my eczema is settling.'

This case illustrates the fact that homeopathic remedies can produce severe aggravations and should be used very carefully. Just because they are so dilute, they are not necessarily harmless.

CASE 35

A 35-year-old woman had suffered from hayfever for eleven years. She was also very sensitive to cats; she only had to go into a room where a cat had been, and within twenty minutes both her eyes and nose were streaming and itching. Allergy tests had confirmed her sensitivity to grass pollens, trees, house dust and cats.

I gave her a mixture of the four allergens in the 30c potency, with instructions to take a dose twice daily whilst she was at risk of exposure to any of these allergens. Two months later she reported that she now had no trouble with cats, and had even spent eight hours in a house where there were three cats, 'without a tickle'.

CASE 36

A 35-year-old man complained that every time he drank any beer he started sneezing and developed a nasal discharge.

Purely empirically (and I can't think for what reason I chose this medicine) I gave him a supply of *House dust mite* 30c, and suggested he took one before each visit to his pub.

He surprised me by reporting, about two months later, that he could now drink 1½ pints of beer with impunity, that the copious production of catarrh for the following four hours had ceased, and that he had regained his sense of smell, which had been absent for the last two years.

In the subsequent twenty years I have repeated this experiment in similar circumstances on two occasions, with the same gratifying results. I am afraid I cannot offer any explanation for this outcome.

Many people become sensitive to articles of daily diet, and an allergy to eggs is not uncommon:

CASE 37

A 63-year-old publisher attended on account of his allergy to eggs, which had developed after a vagotomy ten years previously. Whenever he ate a fried or boiled egg, he developed within the hour severe griping abdominal pains, followed by profuse watery diarrhoea: 'The pain was awful', he said. He could tolerate small amounts of egg custard with minimal discomfort.

I gave him *Whole egg* 30c, to be taken at weekly intervals for four weeks, and then at fortnightly intervals as required. Three months later he insisted that the allergy had literally stopped the same day, and to test this he had taken a challenging dose of boiled egg, without any untoward sequelae. 'This surprised me, as I have eaten boiled and fried eggs too many times over the years to be in any doubt about their effect on me.'

My immediate suspicion was that this unusually quick response was psychosomatic, but the benefit lasted many years. He admitted he was most sceptical at first and had not expected the treatment to work. He had continued taking the tablets, not daring to stop in case he relapsed. I reduced the frequency to monthly doses, and he has been able to enjoy his favourite breakfast once again, without fear of the consequences.

Allergic reactions are becoming more common, and a large group of man-made allergens has come to join the animal, vegetable and mineral categories reported above. These are the organic chemical products used in industry and agriculture – solvents, bleaches, pesticides, preservatives, etc. – which may prove difficult to correlate with the symptoms.

CASE 38

In the days when chlorine was used to disinfect swimming pools, inflammation of the eyes after swimming was a frequent occurrence. In the summer of 1973 I conducted a trial of giving swimmers three doses of *Chlorum* 30c once a week before the swimming session.

One participant reported as follows: 'After each pill I developed sore, running eyes and nose, like hayfever, which lasted for a little while, but now I can stand swimming without any adverse reactions.' She was most impressed.

CASE 39

A 10-month-old boy was admitted to hospital following his first febrile convulsion. Thereafter he had many readmissions on account of twelve further febrile convulsions in the next year. His temperature would rise to 43°C (109.5°F), and the fever lasted on average three to four days, the attacks occurring at approximately two week intervals.

Extensive investigations at the local hospital and the Birmingham Children's Hospital included an intravenous pyelogram, a whole body CAT scan, and urinary catecholamine estimation. All tests were unremarkable, and it was postulated that each episode must be due to an unidentified viral infection. He was routinely medicated with paracetamol, co-trimoxazole, and sodium valproate, which in the opinion of his mother and his GP did not seem to make any significant difference to the course of the attacks or illness.

His mother, a very sensible woman, trained in nursing children with learning difficulties, was able to remain surprisingly calm when these alarming fits occurred. She possessed her own set of homeopathic remedies, but neither *Aconite* nor *Belladonna* were successful in controlling her son's fevers.

On 5.10.81 I wrote to the paediatrician as follows:

'As Russell continued having further pyrexias lasting three to four days, which were not being adequately controlled with paracetamol, I prescribed homeopathic *Pyrogen* (putrid beef), which seemed to fit his symptoms, and which I considered to be worth trying. Mother, reporting today [a month later] says that although he has had four further bouts of pyrexia lasting between two and four days, the homeopathic preparation by itself reduces the temperature to normal after half an hour, and works for about eight hours, during which time Russell seems quite his normal lively self. Incidentally his mother is now far happier with his progress (although he is still having the pyrexias) because he has now caught up on all his developmental milestones, whereas before he seemed to be regressing.'

From that time onwards (September 1981) the fevers were adequately controlled with *Pyrogen* 10M, and paracetamol was

83

withheld. Although his temperature spiked to the region of 40°C (104°F) he did not have febrile convulsions. His hospital investigations were continued, but consistently proved inconclusive; so far no cause for the febrile attacks had been discovered.

It was his mother's perception that solved the enigma. In August 1983 she became convinced that his fevers were associated with his craving for plums and tomatoes, which she had indulged since he was nine months old. She promptly withheld these suspected foods, and the attacks virtually ceased. Later she introduced locally grown plums and tomatoes into his diet, and found he could eat these liberally without any reaction.

On 18.1.84 the paediatrician wrote: 'As you know, Russell is rather better; he has had no further fevers for six months since he has stopped eating foreign plums and tomatoes. He has had no convulsions for ten months, and has stopped his sodium valproate altogether, as it made him very sleepy ... I will review him in a year's time.'

To date [September 1986], he has only had three similar febrile attacks in the last three years, during which time all foreign plums and tomatoes have been excluded from his diet. The first followed eating canned tomatoes, the second occurred after eating local grown tomatoes which, it transpired had been sprayed, and the third was attributed to a food additive. On each occasion he was treated with *Pyrogen* 10M, and had no convulsion, though on one occasion he 'twitched'.

Pyrogen is a medicine I rarely prescribe, presumably because nowadays we rarely see cases of hyperpyrexia due to puerperal pyrexia, septicaemia, typhoid or phthisis. Tyler (*Homoeopathic Drug Pictures*) and Clarke (*Dictionary of Practical Materia Medica*) between them give a full account of its introduction to homeopathic therapeutics. It should be considered as part of the group of medicines which includes *Baptisia*, *Rhus tox.*, *Anthracinum* and *Echinacea*. Like *Baptisia* there is mental confusion, oral foetor, great prostration, myalgia and a tachycardia out of proportion to the rise in temperature; like *Rhus tox.* there is a constant restlessness, but the first movements are not painful.

In future there may be an increasing use for this medicine if food preservatives or additives are found to cause a pyrogen-type of pyrexia in certain sensitive subjects.

CASE 40

Sometimes the cause of the allergic reaction cannot be ascertained, but homeopathic remedies are still effective in treating it. One evening in January 1976 I received a telephone call from the nurse in charge of the geriatric unit attached to our local general hospital. I was then a clinical assistant, and provided emergency cover two nights per week.

An 86-year-old woman had suddenly developed oedema of her tongue, which had swollen rapidly over two hours and was now causing concern. They had no antihistamine injections in the drug cupboard, and the dispensary was closed.

On examination, I found the tongue grossly swollen and filling her mouth. The patient was distressed and uncommunicative. I dissolved about a dozen granules of *Apis mel.* 30c in a glass of warm water, and instructed the nurse to administer teaspoon doses every quarter of an hour. I also left an ampoule of an antihistamine for injection if the swelling did not rapidly subside, and instructions to contact me again if the patient had not improved.

I heard nothing further until I enquired the next morning. Apparently the swelling had resolved soon after I left, and had not returned. The antihistamine injection had not been given.

The constitutional approach to the treatment of allergies is discussed in the next chapter.

Chapter 7

Catarrh, Asthma and other Respiratory Cases

It is a general rule with homeopathic prescribing, that where possible the *constitutional* remedy should be ascertained and given. This is not always as easy as it sounds. Some patients fit very neatly into a 'constitutional' type, others do not. In acute illness a 'warm-blooded' *Pulsatilla* type can alter and become very chilly, and display all the features of a patient who requires *Arsenicum album*.

CASE 41

A middle-aged woman had suffered from catarrh for a year, following a cold. Her nose felt completely obstructed, despite a constantly running watery discharge. Her nostrils burned, and she had lost her senses of taste and smell. Her eyes were not affected. Antihistamine tablets and *Pulsatilla* failed to help, but she had some relief from a nasal spray.

On examination the nasal passages appeared oedematous and blocked, with a watery discharge.

After six doses of *Sabadilla* 12c every two hours, she was able to breathe better than for months, and on examination the inside of the nose was no longer oedematous.

A single dose of *Arsenicum album* 200c was given, and after ten days she could taste and smell for the first time in a year.

Silica is well recognised as a 'catarrhal' remedy, but works even better if it fits the constitutional type.

CASE 42

A 68-year-old man had suffered from nasal catarrh and frontal sinusitis for thirty years. He was a chronic mouth breather and had lost his sense of smell. At times his catarrh was so bad that he would lose his balance too.

He was a chilly person with cold extremities, and always wore a hat or cap when out of doors. A warm atmosphere helped to relieve his catarrh, and in bed at night he found he could breathe better if he pulled the bedclothes over his head. He loved ballroom dancing, but was embarrassed because his head and neck sweated profusely.

I gave him *Silica* 200c to be taken at intervals of two weeks if required. Six weeks later he reported a vast improvement. After a slight initial aggravation, 'I began to improve in about two weeks, and for the last month I have not used a single handkerchief in a day, whereas I used to use a dozen a day.'

He was no longer mouth breathing, and his sense of smell was returning.

He maintained his improvement during the remaining years he kept in touch with me, and did not have a recurrence of his sinusitis. He reduced the frequency of *Silica* to monthly doses, and ultimately stopped taking it altogether.

Silica is a deep and slow-acting medicine, which should only be given infrequently when used in the 200c potency (usually at a minimum of two-week intervals).

Sometimes the patient when questioned will recognise that his illness dates from some shock, accident or severe mental trauma, in which case medicines like *Opium, Arnica, Natrum mur., Staphysagria*, and so on would be indicated. It is interesting to find that Kent, in his *Repertory*, listed medicines to combat the effects of ailments from: anger, disappointed love, grief, reproaches, scorn, and 'mortification' (humiliation). The homeopathic physicians were a century ahead of their colleagues in the understanding and treatment of psychosomatic illness (see Chapter 4).

Nosodes

One also sees children whose hayfever, asthma, eczema, arthritis or other chronic condition originated after a smallpox vaccination, or an infection such as measles. Giving the appropriate 'nosode' often results in a cure of an illness that has resisted years of conventional treatment. A 'nosode' is made from disease products, and the appropriate two for the causes mentioned would be *Variolinum* and *Morbillinum*. If the patient complains that he has never felt well since he had a BCG inoculation, or has a strong family history of tuberculosis, he requires a similar product given back again in potency as *Tuberculinum bovinum*.

A person may suffer from catarrhal symptoms due to some inborn genetic trait, or diathesis, transmitted from his parents or grandparents. A high potency of the appropriate nosode may alter this disposition, and improve or cure him.

CASE 43

A 2½-year-old boy with Down's syndrome suffered from persistent nasal catarrh, for which no treatment had so far been effective. *Thuja*, although well indicated, was not helpful in this case. I therefore used a nosode because of his inborn genetic trait.

I gave him *Medorrhinum* 200c to be repeated at four to fourteen days' interval, according to response. Two years later the mother reported: 'It's been great, the tablets just clear the catarrh in twenty-four hours – nothing has ever done that before. Every two or three months I give a tablet morning and night, never more than three in total, and it's very successful.'

Bowel Nosodes

Certain chronic conditions which improve, but are not cured, when the indicated medicine is given, may need a 'bowel nosode' to complete the recovery. Groups of homeopathic remedies have been found to correlate with certain of the bowel flora, and potencies made from these bacteria can be used to enhance the action of medicines to which they correspond.

CASE 44

A service engineer of forty-five had a four years' history of attacks of incessant sneezing and profuse watery nasal discharge, persisting all the year round. The sneezing was worse in the morning on rising, and usually lasted for half an hour, though sometimes it went on all day, preventing him from going to work. The paroxysms were so violent that on occasions he hurt himself while sneezing. The nasal discharge was profuse, and so clear that his handkerchiefs (several each day) could be squeezed out dry and still appear clean. His nose was blocked between attacks of sneezing, but cleared when he sneezed. There was minimal itching of the eyelids, and minimal reddening and watering of the eyes, and his throat and palate were unaffected. He had lost his sense of smell.

On examination, the mucous membrane of the nose was so injected, tender and swollen that it was impossible to insert a nasal speculum.

He had been fully investigated at hospital four years previously, and allergy tests showed sensitivity to pollen and house dust. A course of desensitising injections had been prescribed, but after the sixth injection he told me, 'I nearly died, as I could not breathe.' So far he had had slight relief only from a multiplicity of antihistamine tablets and nasal sprays.

I prescribed *Sabadilla* 12c, three times a day until reaction.

Two weeks later he phoned to say that he was better, the number of sneezes being much reduced. He got an immediate aggravation after each dose, but then was better for two or three days. I sent him *Sabadilla* 200c, to be taken as required.

A month later he reported, 'The pills worked wonders, my nose has never been so clear.'

A fortnight after the pills ran out the condition relapsed, and he was given one dose of the bowel nosode *Sycotic co.* 10M, after which he continued to improve.

This particular bowel nosode was chosen because of its reputation for alleviating chronic catarrh.

CASE 45

A 5½-year-old boy had suffered from over twenty attacks of acute otitis media in the two years before his first homeopathic consultation, and had had a full course of antibiotics each time. The pain was very severe, and usually lasted seven hours before the drum perforated. The attacks occurred on average once a month, with two weeks' illness alternating with two weeks' health, accompanied by frequent coughs and colds. On one occasion only he had had a three-month remission.

An audiogram revealed hearing loss, and he was on the waiting list for insertion of grommets.

He was warm-blooded and discarded his blankets at night, he had a dry skin, liked company, and had no fears. He liked thunder, he had nasal catarrh, and was not thirsty.

I prescribed:

Tuberculinum 1M in a single dose.

Sycotic co. 30c twice a day, once a week.

Aconite and *Belladonna* 30c to be used as indicated at the beginning of each attack.

Three months later he had only had one attack, and he could then hear whispers. I reduced the *Sycotic co.* to fortnightly doses. Three months later he still had not had an attack, although on several occasions his parents had used *Aconite*, followed by *Belladonna* at the first signs of one. However, he was still getting colds, so I prescribed:

Natrum mur. 30c, four times a day, at the onset of each cold.

Homeopathic 'Influenza and common cold tablets' (a nosode made from influenza and common cold viruses), one a month.

A year later his parents reported excellent progress, with no ear infections, 98% improvement in his hearing, and no need for grommets. However, they were concerned at his lack of self-confidence and anxiety, particularly in the classroom.

I prescribed *Lycopodium* 30c every fourth morning.

Two months later his mother reported that his attitude had changed, and he was far more confident in the classroom.

....

Homeopathic prescribing is a fascinating study that embraces every aspect of the patient, mentally, physically and environmentally, including his past and family history. It may be time-consuming, but the results are highly rewarding, and people who have been successfully treated with homeopathy rarely want to revert to conventional treatment. My next case concerns one of these exceptions.

CASE 46

A few years ago I was telephoned by a consultant who introduced himself as the new chest physician at a certain Midlands hospital. He then said, 'I am amazed and intrigued by your treatment of Mr H. with homeopathic *Pulsatilla* and *Sanguinaria nitrica*.' He went on to observe that he had an open mind about alternative medicine, yet homeopathy had always had an unfavourable write-up in the medical press, and he had never seen any results of controlled trials involving homeopathy. He asked, 'Why had not more trials been conducted? It must be absurd to say homeopathy cannot be verified by trials.' (This conversation took place before the *British Medical Journal* published the article by Dr Kleijnen et al., in which they reported their assessment of 107 controlled trials in 96 published reports of the efficacy of homeopathy in humans (*BMJ* 1991; 302:316–33).

Then reverting to my patient he confided, 'We can successfully treat and control asthma with conventional drugs, that's really no problem, but we cannot touch rhinitis – and here is this man who has had perennial rhinitis for years, and you cured him with homeopathy!' He could have added 'in one consultation', because I had only seen the man once, six weeks earlier, and this was my first feedback as to his response to homeopathic treatment. So what was so intriguing about this case?

The man in question was a headmaster whose daughter I had apparently treated successfully for glue ear some nine years earlier. He was a non-smoker and teetotal. He had suffered from rhinitis for twenty years, was allergic to many substances, including all wines, nylon, and zinc plasters. He had had a nasal polyp removed in 1988, and had reacted badly to the general anaesthetic. A month later he woke in an attack of asthma. (The chest consultant told him that polypectomy was a well-known precipitant of asthma.) The patient now had total loss of smell, and developed annual winter colds, invariably associated with wheezing respiration. He also suffered from nasal catarrh, though not hayfever, and was a mouth-breather, because his 'nose was blocked'. His catarrh was clear mucus, yellow or green, and often blood-streaked.

He felt better after a cool shower: 'It unblocks my nose.'

Because his respirations were so noisy his wife slept in a separate room.

He never developed labial herpes.

He was warm-blooded and slept without pyjamas.

Thirstless: 'I could go all day without a drink.' 'Moist-eyed' when stirred emotionally. He liked fat, but avoided it – though was not particularly upset by it.

He liked excessive salt.

Finally, he had anal irritation, for which he had a local injection, without lasting relief.

He was currently using two metered aerosols:

salbutamol, and
beclomethasone dipropionate

My prescription had been:

House dust 200c single dose
Sulphur 30c twice a day, four doses starting next day

If no significant response after one week:

Pulsatilla 30c on waking, every seventh day as required, and
Sanguinaria nitrica 6c three times a day on intervening days, when not taking *Pulsatilla*.

I didn't see him again for six months, some three months after the consultant had phoned me. He explained that when he had attended hospital for review, 'The physician kept quizzing me about homeopathy, to which I could only reply, You had better ask

Dr Jack that one.' This must have stimulated the consultant to contact me.

His rhinitis certainly had improved remarkably and the improvement had been sustained; however he still had total loss of smell.

I prescribed *Teucrium marum* 3c three times a day until reaction, discontinuing both *Pulsatilla* and *Sanguinaria nitrica. Teucrium* (cat-thyme) has mainly been used to treat threadworm infections which are often associated with the itching anus from which he suffered. *Teucrium* is indicated for nasal polypi with loss of smell, and these were the two residual symptoms from which the patient suffered.

The effect was surprising. He phoned me a week later to say that he had taken *Teucrium* 3c as directed, but after two days had begun to develop thick catarrh. He continued for another three days, and then had to stop because his nose was completely blocked. He felt 'flu-ish' and took to his bed, where he slept for thirty-six hours, waking the third day with his nose clear and his breathing much improved.

Out of curiosity I phoned Mr H. a year later to enquire of his progress, and he had sad news for me. He had enjoyed six months of complete freedom, with ability to breathe through his nose, then the catarrh returned followed by nasal blockage and impeded respiration. He tried the homeopathic medicines again, but without relief. His GP reluctantly started him on oral prednisolone and a steroid nasal spray, and a further polypectomy was performed. He explained that he had not contacted me because he was under the impression that homeopathic medicines were inactivated by steroids, which he knew he still needed, and was taking. In fact, along with other experienced homeopaths, I find that the correct simillimum can still work even though the patient is on systemic steroids, in many cases allowing the dose of pred-nisolone to be reduced gradually and safely by the patient's GP.

This case is interesting because the improvement following homeo-pathic treatment was assessed and recorded by an independent expert who could hardly be accused of bias towards homeopathy. It also illustrated that low potencies (3c) can cause marked aggravations, though this is unusual, especially in such a short time.

I would like to emphasise that I personally, along with many other doctors practising homeopathy, find it advantageous and often necessary to use conventional medicines as well. Modern drugs have a definite place in the treatment of conditions such as asthma and serious infection, and indeed it is imperative that conventional medic-ation is never withdrawn suddenly. Homeopathy will work alongside other drugs, and only if the condition being treated shows a definite improvement should these drugs be carefully reduced, with the co-operation and agreement of the patient's general practitioner.

Another reason that I use conventional medication is that successful prescribing in homeopathy is time-consuming, and when one has a crowded surgery and is pressed, it is impracticable to give the necessary time to every patient to decide which homeopathic remedy they require. If the wrong homeopathic remedy is prescribed because not enough time was taken in the consultation, not only will no benefit ensue, but the patient has been denied the chance of improvement with conventional treatment. Having said that, when it is possible to find the correct homeopathic medicine, it may well be far more effective than its conventional counterpart; or indeed no conventional effective remedy may exist.

....

Homeopathy can be used to treat a broad spectrum of respiratory disease, from persistent cough to whooping cough, from asthma to bronchitis.

CASE 47

Take, for instance, baby Shirley, born on 8th April, 1971, birth weight 2.5 kg (5 lb 9 oz). Her mother had a very rapid and uncomplicated confinement.

Age three weeks: onset of whooping cough.

Pertussis confirmed by paediatrician (baby now aged five weeks). Chlorpromazine syrup 20 ml and tetracycline given. Parents warned of high mortality rate for babies of that age.

13.5.71. *Drosera* 200c (sundew), one dose given. Having attacks of cyanosis, going stiff, choking, etc.

25.5.71. Phlegm thick, tenacious, long and stringy. *Coccus cacti* 6c (cochineal), one dose four times a day given.

2.6.71. Very much improved. *Coccus cacti* continued.

9.6.71. Cough worse again, although baby's general condition good. gaining weight. *Mephitis* (skunk) 1c four times a day given. Complete recovery.

One of the most useful medicines in the list, in my experience, is *Bryonia* (wild hop), so-called because of its rapid growth spurt in the spring, when it 'bursts forth'. This climbing plant covers the hedgerows, clinging on by its tendrils, and has a hairy, ivy-like leaf. Its white flowers are replaced in the autumn by scarlet berries, and it has a very characteristic drug picture.

It attacks all serous membranes, thus affecting the pleura and joints. Its pains are very characteristic, being worse for the slightest movement and better for pressure. The patient wants to be alone, and resents any interference, and is very thirsty for cold drinks. You can remember this by: *BRYONIA* – DRY-alonia! It has a marked intolerance of heat.

CASE 48

In the pre-antibiotic era there was a middle-aged woman who developed a right-sided pneumonia who, when I visited her, was lying very still in bed. She resented my interference, because the least jerk of the bed jarred her and produced her chest pain. She lay very quietly in bed, not daring to take a deep breath, holding her chest with her hand.

When I tried to help her sit up, to examine her chest, she promptly fainted. Her cough racked her and she wanted repeated large drinks of cold water. Her tongue was parched and coated. She had been taking strong analgesic tablets for her pain, but she found *Bryonia* 30c, taken every alternate hour, far more effective. She made a complete recovery.

CASE 49

Herbert was a chronic bronchitic, aged sixty-two years. He had had pneumonitis in 1957 and his chest X-ray appearance in 1958 was: 'Mid-zone regions are fibrotic. There are bronchitic appearances'.

In 1966 his chest X-ray showed 'generalised emphysema and bronchitis and cor pulmonale'.

He had been unable to work since that date. It was as much as he could do to walk one mile along the level to the surgery.

He was maintained on aminophylline, repeated courses of tetracycline, theophylline and ephedrine tablets, and glyceryl trinitrate tablets for his angina.

3.5.68. Attended for a 'sick certificate' and repeat prescription. He had pains in his chest, and his breathing was very bad.

Modalities: Worse wet, worse damp, worse fog, worse cold, chilly, hands feel frozen. Better warm, better dry. Unaffected by wind (unless very cold). Tight breathing, stinging in throat sometimes. Better walking, but some days could not walk at all. Unpredictable, because within an hour of feeling well his chest might 'tighten up' and he could not move freely. Afraid on this account to go into town and frightened to admit feeling well in case situation relapsed. No time aggravation. Liked salt and fats. Smoked moderately until thirty years ago, nil since.

Given *Sulphuric acid* 30c, twice daily for six doses.

13.5.68. Breathing very much better. Chest pains gone. Prescribed *Sulphuric acid* 30c to be taken as necessary.

1.11.68. Further prescription for *Sulphuric acid* 30c, as is beneficial.

CASE 50

A 66-year-old man had suffered from bronchitis for thirty years since stopping smoking. His chest physician, whom he attended regularly, had apparently recently told him to stop all medication, as it was ineffective in his case. (This was before the days of the modern inhalers.)

The patient's main problem was his attacks of paroxysmal coughing, with copious production of tenacious sputum. His colourful description included: 'The cough is choking, horrendous, and wakes me three or four times a night. I have to get up and stand for three quarters of an hour coughing up half a cupful of sticky catarrh. It often makes me vomit, and frequently I have to leave a meal and cough until I am sick. The cough makes me sweat, gives me a headache, makes my eyes water and leaves me very short of breath.'

His condition had deteriorated in the few months before seeing me. He was a chilly man who loved heatwaves, was thirsty, and whose tongue was white. His peak flow rate was 360, against an expected 580.

I prescribed:

House dust 200c in a single dose.

Sycotic co. 30c, 3 doses at 12-hour intervals.

Kali bich. 3c, four times a day, to follow.

A month later he was '50% better', so I increased the potency of *Kali bich.* to 30c daily.

Another month later he was '70% better', and said it was 'unbelievable, and there is definitely far less phlegm.'

However he felt that the 30c of *Kali bich.* had not been as effective as the 3c, so he reverted to the lower potency.

The following month he was able to sleep through the night nine nights out of ten. 'It's a pleasure to lie in bed and breathe comfortably.'

He maintained his improvement through the winter months, despite developing colds, and finally settled on *Kali bich.* 6c three times a day, which he was very reluctant to stop.

Kent's *Repertory* has a special, often overlooked, section on 'Expectoration'. In each of the three rubrics: 'Ropy', 'Stringy', 'Viscid', *Kali bich.* is in bold type. It is also in bold type in the rubric for 'White tongue', in the Mouth section, under 'Tongue, discoloration'.

CASE 51

Mrs J.G. had a cough that was most distressing and embarrassing, the more so because she loved attending her church services three times each week, and she unintentionally announced her presence within minutes of arrival.

The cough was loud, harsh, paroxysmal, suffocative and exhausting, and although she was routinely supplied with a glass of water she could not control the attacks. The bouts recurred at short intervals throughout the whole of the service. She had had the cough for some four months. The climax came one Sunday morning. Her cough was so persistent and disruptive that it made it difficult for anyone to follow the sermon, and it spoiled the tape recording, to which those who were unable to attend would want to listen.

She had had several courses of antibiotics, had been X-rayed and was now under the care of a chest physician, who had diagnosed a viral infection.

On direct questioning she admitted that the cough produced urinary incontinence, which was not surprising. The cough was just as severe all day at home as when in church.

I gave her a few doses of *Causticum* 200c, to be taken at two-hour intervals.

During the evening service she sat in the row behind me and I, and many others in the congregation, noticed the complete absence of her cough during the whole of the service. At the close she leaned forward and tapped my wife, and said to her: 'Wasn't that marvellous?' My wife, who did not know that I had treated her agreed, thinking she was referring to the sermon! The woman then added 'I didn't cough once, although twice I thought it was starting.' Her family, who were present, were 'amazed'. Later I learned that several of the congregation commented among themselves about their surprise and relief that the service had not been interrupted by her cough.

I gave her a prescription for *Causticum* 200c, to be taken as required on the first sign of a relapse. Initially she took daily doses, then one at two to three day intervals, and after two weeks, at weekly intervals. After three months she discontinued treatment, and during the following three years only had to take a few doses of *Causticum* 200c at infrequent intervals.

If the cure was due to homeopathic *Causticum* it was unusually quick for a chronic illness, although this does happen occasionally. In general, the more acute the condition the more speedy the response; chronic conditions respond more slowly.

I did not feel that the cough was of hysterical origin, nor the cure a placebo response; she had not only tried all the current cough linctuses in vogue that she could buy, or her GP had prescribed, but had experimented with several different homeopathic medicines which she obtained from a health shop, all to no avail.

CASE 52

Hilda was an overweight blonde woman of 62 years.

She had had a distressing cough for nearly a month. She had had several strong linctuses containing codeine and methadone but was getting no sleep and was choking with the cough. She was so depressed that the husband requested a visit for her. She started crying the moment I arrived.

She was unable to expectorate and found that sipping water helped a little. She was worse in the warm and had to turn off the central heating.

She had no thirst. I gave her *Pulsatilla* 30c four times a day.

Two days later her husband rang to ask for more pills as they had helped far more than any of the linctuses.

CASE 53

A six-year-old girl attended me in 1957 with repeated epistaxes, at about weekly intervals for two years. She had been seen by an ENT surgeon who could find no sign of trouble in her nose. I gave her *Millefolium* (yarrow) 1c, three times a day for twelve doses, and she then went a full month without a bleed. She then relapsed and had nose bleeds on four consecutive nights, so I gave her a further three-day course of *Millefolium*. Following this she did not have another nose bleed as long as I followed her up, which was ten years.

For cases of epistaxis in the elderly population, particularly in a plethoric person with a bright red face, I find *Melilotus* (sweet clover) most often indicated. The observation that haemorrhage occurred in cattle who had fed on mouldy sweet clover led to the discovery of coumarins, which were developed as anticoagulant drugs. Coumarins prevent the formation of clotting factors, mainly factor 7 and prothrombin, from vitamin K in the liver. Homeopaths had known for nearly one hundred years previously that *Melilotus* was indicated for congestive headaches and a tendency to haemorrhage.

CASE 54

Miss R.L., a land worker aged 43 years, had suffered from asthma all her life.

She was a tall, well-built woman.

15.11.66. She attended after having a bad attack the previous fortnight, with a residual feeling of tightness in her chest. An X-ray ten years previously was clear.

Her attacks were worse at midnight if she went to bed early, otherwise she would wake at 4a.m. in an attack. She had to sit up and lean forward, and was better rocking. She had a productive cough, with white phlegm each morning.

Worse after exposure to dust and in dry weather.

Worse premenstrually. Chilly. Wore polo-necked jumpers. Liked fat; added salt.

She was given *Kali carbonicum*, in a series of potencies, from 30c, 200c, 1M to CM, alternate mornings.

29.11.66. Telephoned to say she was very much improved.

She still woke occasionally at 3a.m. for a short time, and had to sit up and cough.

Aconite 30c sent, to be taken at quarter-hourly intervals in attacks.

28.2.67. Letter received to say that she was very much better. No asthma at all during the day, and only occasionally at night. I sent her six doses of *Kali carb*. 30c to be used if necessary.

CASE 55

A 52-year-old factory machinist developed eczema at 42 years old, and late onset asthma five years later. His asthma rapidly deteriorated so that his chest physician prescribed courses of oral prednisolone, in addition to aminophylline and inhaled salbutamol and beclomethasone. Initially the courses were at three-monthly intervals, then two-monthly, and in the six months preceding his first consultation with me, every three weeks. With this therapy his peak expiratory flow (PEF) was 450, against a target of 600 for his height and age. His consultant had advised him to buy a nebuliser, but his GP apparently had cautioned him against this! He had stopped smoking eight years previously (his father died from asthma at 55 years old, and had smoked all his life). He had no known allergies, but had given away his dog as a precaution. He was always worse in his bedroom, especially on waking, and at weekends when at home, and in the spring.

In my letter to his GP (15.7.91) I fully supported the consultant's recommendation for the patient to obtain a nebuliser and continued: 'I did a skin test to see if he was overtly house-dust mite positive, but the results were unremarkable: this isn't unduly surprising because one obtains false positives and false negatives with this test.'

However, since he is always worse in his bedroom on waking, when his catarrh and asthma are at their most troublesome, I prescribed *House dust* 30c to be taken at intervals of four to fourteen days according to response. I also prescribed *Aconite* 30c, every quarter hour at the onset of acute attacks with palpitations, dyspnoea and distress. I emphasised he must on no account alter his conventional medication, because the homeopathic treatment would work along side it.

Two months later: He had taken his first dose of *House dust* 30c in the evening of the day of his first consultation, and at midnight had had a most alarming attack of asthma. 'It was the worst attack I have ever had in my life. I was stifled and literally couldn't breathe. It was like a seizure – terrible. My wife insisted on calling the doctor, but I stopped her and held on. I thought I was going to die. I couldn't think straight, and forgot all about the *Aconite*. After a while I slowly got my inhaler into me. The attack settled gradually, and I was wheezy all the next day, and I wondered about getting prednisolone from the doctor. It took me a day to realise it was due to the tablet. It must have been – there was no other factor. Since then I've been fine, absolutely fine. My PEF went up to 550 for the next three weeks, and has only gradually returned to 450. The second dose of *House dust* 30c, taken two weeks later, didn't produce any aggravation.'

His mother had died of cancer in the meantime, hence his delay in re-attending, but despite this his asthma had not flared up.

The only problem was that as his chest improved and he stopped his oral steroids, his eczema 'went rampant'. I prescribed *Sulphur* 30c at seven to fourteen day intervals, and *Sulphur* 6c at half-hour intervals when the irritation was severe. He was a hot-blooded hungry *Sulphur* type, who put his feet out of bed at night to cool them.

Two months later I presented him at a meeting of the Midlands Branch of the Faculty of Homeopathy. He repeated the above history, adding, 'Its marvellous. I sleep well now, head down and sleep straight through. I always woke at 2 a.m. for my inhaler, and the first two puffs were difficult, getting the stuff in. Then I woke again at 5 a.m. on week-days, or 6 a.m. at weekends, and got up, because if I lay in, the chest went worse. You have no idea of the relief of going to bed without the fear of waking in an attack. Each morning I used to wake choked with catarrh, now it is minimal.' He felt he was 60–70% better. His eczema was settling.

The consultant had discharged him from the chest clinic. The patient said 'He was so pleased I was stabilised and that my peak flow was excellent, that I hadn't the heart to upset him and tell him about homeopathy. I couldn't knock his legs from under him!' Two months later (9.11.91) his PEF was still 460, and he was sleeping right through each night till 9.30 a.m. on Sundays. He had had two short courses of oral steroids, following heavy colds in the six months since his first attendance.

I reduced his *House dust* 30c to monthly doses, and when last seen two months later he was still improving.

Note

1) Even 30c potencies can have a near fatal aggravation, although it is excessively rare.
2) Usually the more severe the aggravation, the more dramatic the improvement that ensues.
3) The order of cure in homeopathy is from within to without. It is more important to treat and cure the asthma, even at the expense of the eczema, than vice versa.
4) He later needed to replace *Sulphur* with *Petroleum*, and to change the washing powder his wife was using.

CASE 56

Finally, a very difficult case of acute sinusitis took me several attempts at finding a medicine before I hit on the right one. In 1959 a baker's roundsman developed severe sinusitis after an attack of Asian flu. Surgeries were very crowded because of the flu epidemic, and I did not have much time for case taking. First I gave him *Pulsatilla*, then ephedrine nasal drops and codeine, then *Kali bich.*, then *Verbascum* and then *Spigelia*, all to no avail! He himself tried various nose drops and sprays, but the pain was unbearable, worse every morning at 9 o'clock, and was left-sided and affected his left eyeball. On the fifth day the pain was hot and throbbing, so I tried some *Belladonna* 200c, which eased him temporarily, but he was back the following morning at 9 o'clock.

At last I recognised that the periodicity was the important feature, and gave him *Cedron* 30c (rattlesnake bean). The pain lifted entirely in one hour and did not return again to my knowledge during the next few years that he remained on my list. (From Boericke, *Materia Medica*: 'Pain over side of face, coming on at 9 a.m.')

Chapter 8

Cardiovascular Disease

This chapter is a compilation of cases of treatment of cardiovascular disease that illustrate well how effective homeopathy can be in some very difficult cases where conventional medicine was failing to control the disease entirely.

HEART FAILURE

Apis mellifica (Honey Bee)

It is strange how some medicines have come into general use. Just as Withering accidentally discovered the use of the foxglove, which today is still our greatest heart medicine, so some of the most brilliant discoveries in homeopathy were fortuitous. In 1847 in America, a twelve-year-old boy was dying. For three months he had had ascites, a hydrothorax, and suddenly he developed anuria, a hot, dry skin and respiratory and circulatory collapse. A strolling Indian woman suggested giving him a baked honey bee, powdered in syrup. Within twenty-four hours the kidneys were functioning, the temperature subsiding, and the boy made a rapid and complete recovery. The practitioner in attendance was so startled that he described the case, and so *Apis mel.* was included in the homeopathic materia medica. We now know that severe bee stings can produce death immediately by anaphylactic shock, or more slowly by suppression of the kidneys.

Consequently, potentised bee venom can stimulate urinary output in certain cases of renal anuria, even though the patient has failed to respond to all other forms of therapy.

CASE 57

I well remember being called urgently to a man who was dying from acute congestive cardiac failure. It was in February 1965, in the middle of the winter rush and 10 o'clock at night. His history had been a long and interesting one. He was sixty-one years old and employed at a major car factory. He had had hardly a day's illness all his life. In May 1963 he had had a routine chest X-ray at the works which showed dense opacities in the upper left lung. He was referred to a chest unit, where ultimately he had a thoracotomy. As the lesion macroscopically appeared to be a carcinoma, he had a lobectomy performed. However, detailed studies of the frozen section failed to reveal any evidence of malignancy.

In retrospect, he was diagnosed as having had a chronic lung abscess. Despite this, his wound was very slow in healing and three months after his operation he developed an empyema. Accordingly in November 1963 he had a rib resection and drainage of his empyema. Six months later he was still having his wound dressed each day by the district nurse and his drainage tube changed each week at hospital. It was then he began to develop dyspnoea and oedema of his ankles. It was discovered that his albumin-globulin ratio was reversed. He was started on digitalis, oral diuretics and potassium supplements.

Things continued much the same for the next half-year until October 1964, when he required a second drainage operation for his empyema. Following this, he was at long last able to dispense with his drainage tube, and managed to get back to work, still in early congestive cardiac failure. He weathered the following winter, and all went well until the day before the visit I am referring to. He then walked round to my surgery with gross oedema of his legs, which extended up his thighs! As he was already on full doses of digoxin, and already on oral diuretics and potassium supplements, I sent him home for a period of strict bed rest; and it was the next night I had this urgent call.

I found him propped up in bed gasping, slightly cyanosed and very distressed. He had a rattling cough and complained of a burning, stinging pain in his chest. He had no thirst. His oedema now involved his scrotum, which was tense and tender, and measured six inches across. He had not been able to pass urine for ten hours, nor had he the least desire to do so. His bladder, in fact, was neither palpable nor distended. His wife was sure he was dying, and I shared her view.

Because he had been in hospital so many times and was so weary of hospital procedures (remember he had had three operations and sub-sequently had attended every week for well over a year, to have his empyema tube changed), his wife requested that I would respect his wish to be left at home. In any case there was little one could do, even in hospital, now that his kidneys had stopped functioning. Suddenly, the account of the boy dying from renal anuria flashed across my mind and I realised that if ever a man's signs and symptoms cried out for

Apis mel., this man's did. After a preliminary dose of *Aconite*, I gave him a pilule of *Apis mel.* 12c and left him eight more doses to be administered every two hours.

I called next morning to find that after the second pilule he had started passing urine and during the rest of the night had completely filled his commode. He had never previously ever more than half filled it during the night. He was dramatically improved. He was no longer cyanosed, his breathing was easier and his pulmonary oedema cleared. He told me the stinging chest pain had all disappeared four hours after he had taken the first pill. Most spectacular of all was the fact that his scrotal oedema had subsided so much that the skin hung loose and crenated.

I must confess that I had never seen anything similar to this happen in all the eighteen years I had already been in general practice. It was hardly likely to be explicable on psychological grounds. I could have understood it if I had given him an injection, given him oxygen or admitted him to hospital; or even done something which, in his eyes, could have been construed as a life-saving measure. But I had left him at home on a dark winter's night, alone with his frightened wife who firmly believed he was dying; and all I had done was to give him eight sugar pills. He made a good recovery from this episode and returned to work two weeks later. Unfortunately, a month later he developed bronchopneumonia and died in hospital.

HYPERTENSION

CASE 58

H.J., 43 years, first attended for homeopathic treatment on 19.2.75, with a history of severe hypertension and chronic bronchitis. When well he worked at Dunlops as a 'troubleshooter', but had been off work for seventeen months from June 1973 to mid-November 1974. In the last two years he had been admitted to hospital twelve times, on several occasions straight from out-patients, or following an urgent visit by his GP. In that time he had spent twenty-seven weeks in total as an in-patient.

From the hospital discharge letters the following history was abstracted. In 1969 he had had a myocardial infarction and was admitted to an intensive care unit. In July 1973 he was readmitted to hospital with urinary tract infection. His blood pressure was then normal at 150/90. By September 1973 his blood pressure was raised and he was started on methyldopa and oxprenolol. Next month he was again in hospital and the consultant physician reported he had 'haematuria, the passage of a small calculus and the failure of the blood pressure to respond to treatment. He was discharged on very high doses of methyldopa and oxprenolol (2000 mg and 320 mg respectively in 24 hours).'

His only brother had hypertension, and retroperitoneal fibrosis, as a result of which one whole kidney and half of the other kidney had been removed. His father died aged 39 years of 'kidney trouble'.

He continued to be seen in out-patients regularly, and had to have his medication changed and increased on several occasions. He had two bouts of 'micturition syncope', and also attacks of severe headache and dizzy spells. His driving licence was revoked.

A hospital letter on 6.1.75 noted he suffered from occasional episodes of tinnitus, lasting a few seconds only, and bouts of palpitations, but otherwise he remained, in general, well. He also remained hypertensive – blood pressure 200/120 lying and 200/130 standing. 'As this man's hypertension is notoriously resistant to treatment I was unable to suggest any further adjustments to make to his regime, and therefore advised him to continue on the same.'

His last hospital letter, from the department of nephrology, prior to his attending for homeopathic treatment, was on 31 January 1975 when his blood pressure was 180/130 sitting and 170/120 standing. His conventional hypotensive medication was continued at maximum dosage.

19.2.75. First attendance: The patient had an untidy-looking, somewhat dishevelled, swarthy appearance. His facial skin was dry and coarse, his lips were chapped, and he looked tense. He was 1.68 m (5 ft 6 in) tall and weighed 65.8 kg (145 lb). He had been a heavy cigarette smoker until he gave up smoking six years ago. His complaints were very clear-cut:

1) Attacks of bumping, pounding headaches, associated with tunnel vision.
2) Profound lassitude. Unable to do any physical work for the last two years.
3) Feeling very anxious.
4) Recurrent attacks of bronchitis.
5) He was 'hot-blooded', and often slept with his feet out of bed, and with nothing on. He could not stand excessive warmth at home or at the office.
6) He admitted being a suspicious person.
7) He was an extrovert who liked company.

8) He felt worse between 4p.m. and 9.30p.m. each day.
9) His skin was dry.
10) He preferred hot food and drinks.
11) He had a craving for sweets.
12) His appetite was very poor.
13) Yet a small amount of food satisfied him.
14) He had an excessive thirst.
15) A craving for salt.

These last four symptoms are suspect, from a homeopathic prescribing point of view, as they could well be iatrogenically induced. This was certainly confirmed in respect of number 15 above by the fact that subsequently, within a few days of his discontinuing all conventional therapy, his salt craving disappeared completely. He always had had a craving for sweets prior to his illness. Even his anorexia and easy satiety could be attributed to his treatment, because on enquiry he agreed he had previously had a hearty appetite. This illustrates the need to sift the symptoms and eliminate those that are due to the effects of treatment, and are not true individual reactions of the person to his illness.

Hahnemann taught that 'the more general and undefined symptoms: loss of appetite, headache, debility, restless sleep, and so forth, demand but little attention when of that vague and indefinite character, if they cannot be more accurately described; as symptoms of such a general nature are observed in almost every disease, and from almost every drug.'

The symptoms that rank as most important in deciding on the remedy are the mentals: anxiety, suspicious, extrovert. Next in order are the general symptoms: worse for heat, worse between 4p.m. and 9.30p.m., and lassitude. On questioning, the lassitude was not 'aggravation from mental exertion', but a general symptom 'aggravation from physical exertion'. The particulars come last: dry skin, chapped lips, thirst, poor appetite, food preferences, cravings, aversions, etc.

The two medicines that came through each rubric (list of remedies) and competed strongly were *Lycopodium* and *Sulphur*. Abstracting these from the appropriate rubrics in Kent we find:

Anxiety	LYC.	SULPH.
Suspicious	LYC.	SULPH.
Warmth aggravation	LYC.	SULPH.
Evening aggravation	LYC.	SULPH.

Worse 4–8 p.m.	LYC.	SULPH.
Aggravation from physical exertion	LYC.	SULPH.
Dry skin	LYC.	SULPH.
Chapped lips (under 'face')		SULPH.
Desires hot food (stomach)	*Lyc.*	–
Desires hot drinks	*Lyc.*	*Sulph.*

As already mentioned, his craving for salt proved a 'red herring'. Similarly, his extreme thirst could probably be attributed to the diuretics, hypotensives, beta-blockers and tranquillisers he was taking; were this not so, both medicines would still have qualified.

Thirst – extreme	*Lyc.*	SULPH.

Although 'extrovert' is not listed, 'desire for company' would cover part of the symptom. Kent lists *Lycopodium* in heavy capitals, but places *Sulphur* in italics under 'aversion for company'. It is worth noticing that the symptom 'Anxiety' when unqualified, i.e. not localised to certain times, circumstances or situations, is of little use in repertorising as there are nearly forty heavy black entries in this rubric, which contains approximately two hundred remedies!

Taking into consideration the patient's appearance, I considered *Sulphur* to be his constitutional remedy, although I would expect *Lycopodium* would be able to help him, and might be indicated in the future. Kent advises that *Lycopodium* should never be given immediately after *Sulphur*, as *Sulphur* belongs to a rotating group: *Sulphur*, *Calcarea carbonica*, *Lycopodium*. Personally I would only follow *Sulphur* with *Calcarea* if the patient, on subsequent attendance, showed new symptoms that indicated he had changed to need *Calcarea*, the most obvious being that he had become chilly, sweaty, and intolerant of the cold.

Another good reason for choosing *Sulphur* was that it is often indicated at the beginning of the homeopathic treatment of a patient with chronic illness who has previously had heavy medication with conventional medicines, or where there is a paucity of symptoms to prescribe on.

The problem was compounded by the fact that he was suffering from a life-endangering malignant hypertension, was taking maximum doses of drugs, and there was a real risk that if he were to discontinue these in any significant amount his blood pressure would go out of control again, as it had done on so many previous occasions. At all costs he wanted to be able to continue attending work, which he was only just managing to do, and to keep out of hospital.

Various questions presented themselves. How could a homeopathic potency be expected to work whilst he continued to take twenty-one tablets a day? How safe would it be, or fair to him, to withdraw any, or all, of his routine medication, so as to give the potentised *Sulphur* a fair chance to work? How fair would it be to his GP or consultant to alter his medication to any significant extent? Would a high potency produce a vicious aggravation, and if so, in what way? He lived over twenty miles away and I could not be responsible to visit him in the event of any untoward reaction occurring. I adopted the typically British attitude of compromise! His prescription was:

Continue all his present medication, but also take:

3 x *Sulphur* 200c that day – 19.2.75
Belladonna 200c every 15 minutes for headaches in attack
Spartium scoparium φ (broom), 5 drops in water four times a day.

Where serious pathology exists, and the homeostatic response is compromised, low potencies are to be preferred to high. However, in this case, since he was a *Sulphur* patient and since his headache was such a typical *Belladonna* headache, I felt confident in giving him the 200c potency. In many cases, if the 30c potency is effective, a higher potency – up to 200c – will work even better. (Some patients do not respond so well to remedies above 200c.)

The *Belladonna* was only expected to afford temporary relief, as it is a short-acting medicine that needs a deeper-acting medicine to follow it (often *Calcarea carbonica*). As to the simultaneous use of *Spartium*, this was one of the rare occasions when I felt polypharmacy was justified.

On 26.3.75 the patient reported that he was feeling dramatically improved, after the first week. His blood pressure was 150/98 sitting, and 130/100 standing. His ECG was satisfactory, and the serum urea, creatinine and electrolytes were normal. The patient was allowed to resume driving. Even more dramatic was the way the *Belladonna* 200c aborted his pounding headaches. He insisted they 'worked within seconds', and that after the first week he had not had to take any. He was advised to continue his conventional tablets, reducing the propranolol only at the rate of 40mg every third day. He was given *Belladonna* 10M to try in place of *Belladonna* 200c if he got another congestive headache, and a further supply of *Spartium* φ.

16.4.75. Despite my advice, he had stopped all his conventional medication with the exception of hydrochlorthiazide (a diuretic). He had only dared tell his wife about this the previous day. He had not had a single headache in that time and felt very well. His blood pressure at his works surgery the day before had been 130/100, but today was 200/120 settling to 155/110.

Treatment

1 x *Sulphur* M
Spartium φ 15 drops four times a day, and hydrochlorthiazide 100 mg once daily.

8.7.75. Blood pressure 150/115, very tense. Pressures at work very exacting.

Treatment

1 x *Lycopodium* 200c
Spartium φ 15 drops four times a day, and hydrochlorthiazide 100 mg once daily.

His blood pressure continued to decrease slowly, but steadily on this regime. He needed occasional doses of *Belladonna* 10M, *Lycopodium* 200c or *Sulphur* 200c.

He was last seen on 8.3.78, when his blood pressure was 140/105.

Discussion

Concerning this case history, it is at once admitted that an isolated anecdotal account of a single patient is of no statistical significance whatsoever, but some interesting points emerge.

Belladonna is a short-acting medicine which has dramatically eased congestive throbbing headaches in hypertensives with startling rapidity. His description of 'immediately', 'within seconds' is only reiterating what one has heard again and again in similar situations, and gives support to the theory that the medicine is absorbed through the buccal mucosa. The alternative explanation, that the effect is psychological, is unlikely because other homeopathic medicines did not produce this result. A double-blind evaluation study of the effects of *Belladonna* in congestive hypertension headaches could be a useful research project. When this patient had a severe headache his face never resembled that of classic *Belladonna* poisoning. It never actually looked red, but his wife could always tell he had one by the dilation of his superficial temporal arteries and slightly flushed appearance.

The hypotensive effect of *Spartium* tincture does not depend on the homeopathic principle. Its therapeutic action in material doses is thought to be due to its active principal, sparteine sulphate. The effect of this alkaloid of broom is to cause lowering of the systolic and diastolic pressures of the provers, and slowing of the heart rate. In the older editions of Martindale's *Extra Pharmacopoeia* it is included with adonis, convallaria and crataegus, under the heading of 'some other drugs with cardiac action'. There it states 'Sparteine lessens the irritability and conductivity of cardiac muscle, diminishing the frequency and amplitude of its contractions, and has been used in the treatment of tachycardia and functional palpitation. Small doses stimulate and large doses paralyse the autonomic ganglia.'

This last statement is an excellent illustration of the Arndt-Schultz Law, which is the bedrock on which homeopathy rests. (This law states that high doses kill, medium doses inhibit, and small doses stimulate.) The sustained control of this patient's hypertension would appear to depend, in part at least, on *Spartium*, as he has demonstrated on several occasions that reducing the dose, or withholding the medicine, is quickly followed by a relapse.

On many occasions previously and since, I have failed to control severe hypertension (even less severe than in this patient) using *Spartium* alone. I have occasionally succeeded in weaning the patient off methyldopa, bethanidine, or guanethidine, substituting *Spartium* instead, but leaving him on a mild diuretic. It would seem necessary to find and give the patient's constitutional homeopathic medicine; in mild cases of hypertension this is sufficient on its own, without the need for *Spartium* (or a diuretic) as an adjuvant.

Following his first dose of *Sulphur*, the patient's blood pressure dropped dramatically before he was taking the amount of *Spartium* that subsequently proved to be his maintenance dose, and whilst still taking his heavy doses of conventional hypotensives. The author has repeatedly verified that the correctly selected homeopathic medicine will frequently work to a certain extent, despite the patient being on full doses of conventional medicines (e.g. in hayfever, when the patient is taking therapeutic doses of antihistamines; or in arthritis, when the patient is on full doses of analgesics or antirheumatic medication). This is reassuring for the beginner, who need not insist that the patient stops all of his present therapy whilst he cautiously tries his homeopathic prescription. Obviously, the simillimum given in its very small dose is far more likely to be able to stimulate the body defences if those same defences are not being depressed by conventional medication.

Using *Sulphur*, in potency, and *Spartium* alone, the blood pressure has remained at an acceptable level and there have been no observable side effects. Contrast the frequent hospital admissions and months of in-patient treatment, the micturition syncopes, the inability to work or drive a car, the headaches, and the loss of libido, which were experienced when he was on conventional therapy. In one sense the patient is his own control. Under his former therapeutic regime his blood pressure was 'uncontrollable'. Since changing to homeopathic treatment he remained symptom-free, with an acceptable blood pressure, in a most strenuous job for the following two years.

As a direct result of this patient's improvement, both his own GP and his GP's partner started using homeopathy and attended the tutorials in Birmingham regularly. Their local chemist started stocking homeopathic medicines.

PAROXYSMAL ATRIAL TACHYCARDIA

CASE 59

Mrs A.H., age 72.

11.3.76. Suffering from blackouts following attacks of paroxysmal tachycardia for the past three years, worse for the last three months. Happens three to four times per week, but recently three to four times per day, maximum twelve attacks in 24 hours. Gets a few seconds warning of a choking feeling in the throat, burning sensation in the ears and head, before losing consciousness.

On conventional medication including digoxin, a beta-blocker and a tranquilliser.

BP 150/90, apex 70.

All medication stopped except digoxin. Given *Aconite* when necessary and *Iberis* (candytuft) 1c.

19.3.76. No improvement. Two very severe attacks.

Given *Lycopus virginicus* 12c (bugleweed) three times a day until improvement, then sac lac twice a day.

9.4.76. Very much better. Only three blackouts in three weeks. Still occasional palpitations but only mild.

28.5.76. Still getting three or four attacks a week, but not so severe and shorter in duration.

Treatment

Lycopus 30c, single dose only after each attack.

25.2.77. Relapse. Palpitation attacks coming worse even when sitting at rest, or lying in bed.

Treatment

Spigelia 6c (pink-root) three times a day until reaction.

20.5.77. *Spigelia* very effective, takes one daily.

Discussion

Lycopus lowers the blood pressure and reduces the heart-rate. I have mainly used it in treating auricular fibrillation associated with thyrotoxicosis. It is also indicated for treating palpitation with praecordial oppression, due to nervous or emotional causes.

Spigelia is a most useful and effective medicine in treating certain types of migraine, facial neuralgia, and violent attacks of palpitation.

As so often happens in homeopathic treatment, the first effective homeopathic medicine may modify or alleviate the symptoms to such a degree that it is no longer the simillimum. A different medicine is then needed to continue or complete the treatment.

CARDIAC DYSRYTHMIA

CASE 60

On 17.6.88 Mr M.K. consulted me for homeopathic treatment to control his attacks of palpitations, which had distressed him for the last six years. He was an otherwise healthy, active man, a keen fisherman who love walking and hill-climbing. He was 78 years old, 1.72 m (5 ft 8 in) tall and weighed 63.5 kg (140 lb), and smoked on average one small cigar daily.

The attacks of palpitations were unpredictable and lasted between five minutes and four days. They occurred approximately twice every twenty-four hours, mainly when in bed at night, frequently at about 3 a.m. Sleeping with high pillows appeared to lessen the frequency of them. He also suffered from dyspepsia, which often precipitated an attack: he found antacids eased his indigestion, but he could not 'eat a good meal any longer'.

He had been prescribed various different tablets, none of which had helped.

He seemed rather tense and nervous; understandably these episodes caused him considerable anxiety.

I prescribed:

Aconite 30c at five-minute intervals at onset of attacks until improvement.

Iberis 1c, four times a day as long as he was having attacks of tachycardia.

Nux vomica 30c, four times a day, during attacks of dyspepsia.

On 24.10.88, over four months later, his daughter reported: 'I can't believe it. He has only had two attacks since he saw you, and he used to have two attacks a day.'

Comment

Iberis is prepared from a tincture made from the seeds of bitter candytuft, and is one of the many medicines introduced into homeopathy by Hale. The cardiac symptoms of the drug are very pronounced and include:

- Cardiac dyspnoea
- Palpitations with vertigo and choking in the throat
- Waking with palpitations at about 2 a.m.
- Pulse full, irregular and intermittent
- Extreme nervousness and fright

VARICOSE VEINS

CASE 61
Mrs J.M. age 38.

26.11.73. Calves of both legs heavy and ache one week premenstrually for several years. Veins engorged and go brilliant red (also painful piles).

Treatment

Hamamelis 3c (witch hazel) every two hours until improvement.

9.2.74. Requests repeat. 'Marvellous, removes all aching, engorgement and reddening.'

CASE 62
A 50-year-old woman complained that for two years her right leg was sore and ached. She had developed phlebitis in it after her confinement

fourteen years earlier, following which she developed varicose veins. 'For the last two years it's been miserable, with my painful swollen hard veins, but I didn't worry too much until my ankle swelled and went black.' Her GP had prescribed some tablets (? diuretics) which she had not yet used; she wanted to try homeopathy first.

I prescribed *Calc. fluor.* 6c four times a day. (See Boericke, 'Circulatory Organs'.) Six weeks later she returned and said 'The tablets have taken all the swelling out of my ankle, and the soreness. The veins have gone down and my leg is comfortable. The veins are quite soft again; they had been lumpy and hard where I had had the phlebitis. It's marvellous how they have gone down in the time.' She had not yet taken her GP's tablets – 'They are still in the cupboard.'

She said her veins were still improving, and she had reduced the frequency of her medication, because she forgot at times to take the tablets, and 'in any case it said on the bottle "when necessary".'

Normally I encourage patients to take the medicines their GP or consultants have ordered, as I have repeatedly verified that conventional medicines do not antidote homeopathic remedies; homeopathy can effectively be an additional form of therapy.

PERIPHERAL CIRCULATORY DEFECT

CASE 63
The patient was a 48-year-old electrician who had suffered from chilblains and poor circulation all his life. For the last five years his condition had steadily deteriorated. Both his feet and hands were affected, particularly his fingers, which went numb with the cold. Every winter, without exception, he developed chilblains. He was employed mainly in wiring factories and unoccupied buildings, which usually were unheated, and he often had to manipulate fine multicore wires, such as are used by British Telecom. The coldness and numbness of his fingers made this impossible, so that annually he had to stop working for the duration of each cold spell, on some occasions for as long as two months at a time. Within minutes of leaving his warm house and getting into his car his fingers went numb with cold, despite his wearing thick woollen lined gloves. This is typical of Raynaud's disease.

He did not smoke, nor work with vibratory tools. Five years previously he had been fully investigated and had been offered cervical and lumbar sympathectomy, as no medical treatment had relieved his condition. He was taking a conventional vasodilator, which he thought 'helped a little'.

On 1.11.85 he presented as an otherwise fit man, 1.75 m (5 ft 9 in) tall, and 70 kg (154 lb) in weight. His eyes were blue and he had flaxen hair. He was a chilly person who felt the cold keenly; he much preferred hot weather to cold, liking heatwaves best, when he could sunbathe. The only other significant homeopathic clue he offered was that he preferred savoury to sweet foods. On direct questioning he stated his hands were dry; on shaking hands with him they were distinctly cold and moist! His wife, who was with him, confirmed that that was their usual state. He was normotensive (BP 115/65), with a resting pulse rate of 65.

I suggested he tried taking a diet rich in fish oils, and also gave him *Silica* 30c three times for one day, every two weeks, with *Calc. phos.* 3c twice a day on intervening days. On 10.1.86 he reported:

'There has been a 60% improvement already. My fingers no longer go dead within minutes of getting into my car, and I only need to wear thin gloves when driving. I have not felt frozen in this cold weather, my whole body feels warmer. I feel a definite improvement after each 'booster' dose (*Silica*). It works within a couple of days and lasts until the next dose, and then I get a further improvement.'

Treatment

Stop the vasodilator.
Proteus 12c three times for one day, and continuing with
Silica 30c every two to four weeks, as required.
Calc. phos. 3c twice a day on intervening days.

Proteus is a bowel nosode which was added initially into the treatment regime because of its benefit in conditions caused by spasm of the peripheral circulation. (See *The Bowel Nosodes* by Dr John Paterson.)

8.3.86. He had had a relapse in Tenerife during the end of January and the beginning of February. He had not taken his homeopathic tablets with him, as he was visiting a warmer climate. He attempted sea bathing, but the cold water caused his fingers to go numb. Later he went up a mountain to an altitude of 1200 metres (3900 ft) and the cold again precipitated numbness of his fingers. Since returning home and resuming his tablets he had had no relapse, and kept working during the following four weeks' freeze-up, which the weather experts described as 'the coldest February in England for eighty years'. He did not develop any chilblains either!

Treatment
> *Proteus* 10M, 1 dose.
> Continue *Silica* and *Calc. phos.*

22.6.87. 'I had a good winter despite the cold spell. I was able to go shooting in the morning in the coldest of weather. I have had no chilblains since I started taking homeopathic medicines.'

Discussion

His improvement was unlikely to be solely attributable to his fortifying his diet with fish oils, as he got tired of this diet and discontinued it as soon as his condition improved. When he withheld his homeopathic medicine his symptoms returned. I did not ascertain which of the two medicines was responsible for his improvement, though I felt it was predominantly *Silica*. The patient was reluctant to stop taking either, during cold spells, in case of relapse (which involved being off work).

He was a typical *Silica* type, i.e. flaxen hair, blue eyes, chilly, intolerant of cold and draught, worse in the winter, better in warm weather, better for warmth generally and locally, cold clammy hands and feet. He had, however, certain *Calc. phos.* features: chilly, cold extremities, with cold numb feelings, worse for cold weather, better in warm weather and in the summer, and preferred savoury foods. He noticed that most improvement followed each fortnightly dose of *Silica*, which was in the 30c potency, but then the low potency *Calc. phos.* 3c, taken three times daily, would only be expected to produce a gradual, less noticeable benefit. It may well be that both medicines were working, and so I continued with both.

The reason why *Secale* was not prescribed is because it was not indicated. *Secale* produces profound vascular changes, similar to those in scleroderma and Raynaud's disease, and is often indicated in treating these conditions. But it also produces a marked intolerance of external warmth. The patient may objectively feel icy cold, as in hypothermia, but wants to be uncovered and in the cold air; this was the exact opposite of this patient's modalities.

Chapter 9

Gastrointestinal Disease

Homeopathic medicines can complement the management of many diseases of the gastrointestinal tract, ranging from diarrhoea and vomiting in children to colitis and Crohn's disease.

VOMITING AND DIARRHOEA

When children are vomiting it is not only distressing for them but also for their parents, who often feel helpless, wishing they knew what they could do or give to alleviate the child's misery. They may even have a haunting fear that the child may have developed a serious condition such as meningitis or something that requires surgical intervention. Obviously, full assessment by a physician is required if the parents are anxious, but the administration of a medicine from the Home Remedy Kit can often alleviate the distressing symptoms very rapidly – 'before the doctor comes'.

In homeopathic treatment, we are looking for a drug that in toxic doses will predictably produce vomiting, when administered to healthy individuals, and with the same 'modalities'.

Modalities are those factors that qualify a particular symptom: e.g. vomiting associated with thirst for cold drinks or hot drinks, or with diarrhoea, etc., and according to the patient's symptoms.

Kent's *Repertory* is a classified list of symptoms, with the drugs that can cause them. It includes a list of the drugs that cause vomiting, and which thus could be used therapeutically; of the 177 listed, 29 are in bold type, indicating that they are the most effective and most commonly indicated ones for use. But even reducing the number from 177 to 29 leaves a bewildering number of options, and generally only the right medicine will work. However, once we introduce the modalities of the case the task is simplified. For example, if the vomiting is due to ice cream, the rubric only contains four remedies: *Arsenicum album, Calc. phos., Ipecacuanha, Pulsatilla.*

116

Alternatively, if the patient is vomiting bile in the morning, the rubric only lists eight remedies, all in small type except *Sepia*, which is in bold type; and which understandably is one of our best remedies for the morning sickness of pregnancy.

So what are the homeopathic medicines that are most useful in treating an uncomplicated case of gastritis in children? By uncomplicated I am considering a child who has persistent vomiting, without any other localising signs or symptoms to suggest some sinister pathology, such as meningism, headache, neck stiffness and photophobia; or features suggestive of a surgical cause as mentioned previously.

I would nominate *Arsenicum album*, *Ipecacuanha* and *Phosphorus* as the most useful medicines for vomiting, and they are included in the Home Remedy Kit.

Administration

The most acceptable way to administer these medicines is to crush the pills first, and then dissolve them in a little water. The liquid can then either be sipped or given from a teaspoon at frequent intervals.

During the years, I have come to the conclusion that at least 80% of cases of acute gastritis have responded to one of these three medicines; and because each family has a set of these 'home remedies', I have been spared hundreds of daytime visits and dozens of night calls.

Again and again parents have reported that they were about to send for a visit when they remembered their set of medicines, gave the appropriate one, and the child quickly got better. Frequently they would bring the child to the following morning surgery just to check that the improvement was complete, and that there were no sequelae needing further treatment.

Arsenicum album

Arsenicum album is perhaps best known for its use in gastroenteritis, where the patient is chilly, prostrated, and has sickness and diarrhoea simultaneously. The onset often is around midnight; the patient tries to get out of bed to go to the toilet and is surprised to find how weak he feels. Having got there, the persistent diarrhoea may necessitate his staying there a long time, during which he is distressed and embarrassed by repeated attacks of vomiting, when he has no container available for the vomit.

If you are away from home, the most convenient place to have a daytime attack of this sort is on British Rail, provided a toilet is vacant!

The conventional treatment, apart from injections, is to wait until one end or other of the alimentary tract is clear, and then medicate, i.e., if the vomiting stops first, give tablets, if the diarrhoea, then a suppository can be inserted. With homeopathic treatment there is no need to wait, and in such situations a few granules of *Arsenicum album* can be taken dry on the tongue, with dramatic results. It can be equally effective in treating diarrhoea caused by viral or bacterial infections, contaminated foods or watery fruits.

I remember once having to visit a man who had collapsed at the onset of an attack of diarrhoea and vomiting, and I put about ten granules of *Arsenicum album* 30c on his tongue. I called back a few hours later to find him very much improved. He greeted me with 'Isn't sugar a wonderful medicine, Doctor?' In acute conditions the main indications for using *Arsenicum album* include anxiety, restlessness and prostration with chilliness.

The patient wants his body warm, but his head in cool air. (Blankets to the chin, the head out of the window.)

Burning pains, eased by applied heat.

Richard Hughes, more than a hundred and twenty years ago, stated in his *Manual of Pharmacodynamics* that if he were only allowed two homeopathic medicines he would choose *Aconite* and *Arsenicum album*.

Arsenicum album has been successfully used in treating malaria, cholera and typhoid where the symptoms have looked like arsenic poisoning. For the same reason, certain selected cases of hayfever, rhinitis, headaches and many other conditions respond well to this medicine.

CASE 64

An urgent call came at 1.30 a.m. from a man whose wife had woken at midnight with acute colic and simultaneous diarrhoea and vomiting, since when she had fainted three times. 'I felt as if I was going to die, and I still feel like it, and I am cold, so cold ...'

She was given *Arsenicum album* 200c in water, sips every ten minutes. The sickness and diarrhoea stopped completely by 2 a.m., though she still felt very weak and did not want to be left alone.

CASE 65

A couple, newcomers to the district, asked to be included in my practice. The wife, who was diabetic, was subject to recurrent attacks of diarrhoea with vomiting which at times were severe enough to cause her to faint. They occurred about every three weeks, without any obvious precipitating cause, and her previous doctor had found that the only way to control them was with an antiemetic injection. No other form of treatment so far had aborted or controlled the attacks. I referred her to hospital. All tests were unremarkable and a diagnosis was made of either recurrent viral infections or food intolerance, but no further treatment was offered.

Partly in self-defence, I looked for a homeopathic medicine which would cut short the attacks before a doctor's visit became imperative. The symptoms matched white arsenic poisoning so well that I prescribed for her, on the National Health Service, a bottle of granules medicated with *Arsenicum album* 30c, with the usual label: 'Ars.Alb. SICKNESS AND DIARRHOEA GRANULES. When sickness and diarrhoea simultaneously, feeling very cold, exhausted, cannot rest. Burning pains in stomach. Thirst for warm drinks. Cannot bear sight or smell of food. 10 granules in warm water every quarter hour until relief.'

I told her husband to give her one dose as soon as he got the medicine, and then follow the instructions on the label at the onset of each attack. The bottle would contain well over a thousand doses of medicine.

I saw very little of her for three and a half years, and then she brought the empty bottle, with a request for a repeat. She gave me a graphic description of what the attacks had been like, and I said, 'But you haven't sent for me once in the three years since you registered with me.' 'No,' she replied, 'thanks to these sugar grains. They're wonderful, they're marvellous. I just put some on my tongue the moment I start vomiting, and the attack stops, and the whole thing passes over. Mind you,' she added, smiling rather sheepishly, 'I take more than the dose. I take more than ten granules at a time.' It was my turn to smile, and I pointed out to her that, in homeopathy, success doesn't depend on the quantity of the medicine you take. It is hard to understand why; but if each granule is thoroughly medicated, a single granule would work as well as a handful of granules. Probably they are absorbed through the mucous membrane of the inside of the mouth, and the smallest dose will work.

I felt a wave of gratitude to Samuel Hahnemann for discovering the principle of homeopathy, and thought of all the night visits I had been spared.

Ipecacuanha

For persistent nausea, with or without vomiting, with a clean tongue and much saliva. The onset is violent.

CASE 66

The senior practice secretary, aged 62 years, suddenly started vomiting one night at 10p.m. She said, 'I felt queasy, and had to run. The vomiting started and went on, and on, and on, and my abdominal pain was the worst pain I have ever had. I kept returning to the bathroom so often that in the end I took up residence there at midnight. There was no diarrhoea, but I was salivating excessively, and the nausea hadn't eased by being sick. I went very cold.

At 3.30a.m. my husband thought about *Ipecacuanha* in the home remedy set. I took a dose, and after ten minutes the pain disappeared. I was surprised as I expected it might take an hour or so. I no longer felt sick, and wasn't sick again – it was just a miraculous thing. It took me sometime to get warm in front of the gas fire; I had been three and a half hours in the bathroom. I got to bed at 4a.m. The most surprising thing is that when I woke at 8a.m. I felt absolutely fine – as if nothing had happened to me. I got up, feeling fit, and came to work as normal.'

It is not well known that *Ipecacuanha*, in its provings, produces gastralgia, as well as nausea and vomiting.

Clarke, in his *Dictionary of Practical Materia Medica*, describes the pain as 'horrid and indescribable'. It certainly was in her case.

Phosphorus

Gastritis with craving for cold drinks, which are vomited immediately.

Other Medicines

There were some disturbing cases that did not respond to *Arsenicum album*, *Ipecacuanha* or *Phosphorus*; it was then necessary to prescribe another medicine and the two most commonly used in such cases were *Aethusa* and *Veratrum album*, amongst others.

Aethusa cynapium (Fool's Parsley)

This herb was so called either because fools mistook it for the culinary herb or because, if eaten in excess, it resulted in inability to think, or fix the attention. Larger doses caused thought blocking, irritability, anguish, crying and even hallucinations. It also produced a marked intolerance of milk and a virulent form of diarrhoea and vomiting, especially during heatwaves. The symptoms developed with alarming rapidity, leading to dehydration and collapse, a pale face with a whitish-blue pallor around the mouth, sweating and vacant staring. It was used extensively in past generations for the fulminating and often fatal forms of infantile gastroenteritis known as 'cholera infantum'.

Kent in his *Materia Medica* graphically described the situation: 'Death is stamped on the face from the beginning, and if there is any remedy in the book that saves life this is one of them.'

The following three case histories illustrate my own experiences of the power of *Aethusa* in potency:

CASE 67
Sarah, age 19 months
Sarah developed severe diarrhoea and vomiting during a heatwave. She was fractious and miserable.

By the third day her mother called me in – 'I have been up all night with her, nursing her and trying to get her to settle.' She had been very hot, but now was collapsed, clammy, and dehydrated. She was vomiting everything, including boiled water.

Her mother had already tried *Arsenicum album* and *Phosphorus* from their home remedy kit to no avail. I felt I had no option but to admit her, but her parents were reluctant and begged me to try something else first. I gave the mother some *Aethusa* 200c in granule form, to be administered every hour, on the strict understanding that I would admit Sarah to hospital in two hours if there was not a marked improvement in that time.

The following day, her mother brought Sarah to the surgery. She was delighted – the baby had not vomited or had diarrhoea since the first dose. After the second dose she slept restfully for five hours (the first time for forty-eight hours) then woke, very much improved, and started to eat and drink, retaining all.

CASE 68

Caroline, age 2 years

She had had diarrhoea and vomiting for twenty-four hours and had not kept any fluid down at all. She had not passed urine for twelve hours and neither *Arsenicum album* nor *Phosphorus* had helped. Her father collected some antiemetic suppositories from morning surgery at 10 a.m. By the afternoon the parents phoned as they were very worried. (Both were trained nurses.) The child was worse and was now dehydrated, hiccuping, and staring vacantly. Urgent hospital admission was arranged, but the father asked me if there was anything else she could take in the meantime. I gave some *Aethusa* 30c, to be given in water every ten minutes.

An hour and a half later the parents phoned me. They had delayed taking her in as she began to improve after the first dose! I promptly visited her to assess the situation; she was obviously much better, had only vomited once in the interim, and was retaining sips of water. I arranged two-hourly phone reports.

The next day they reported that she had had a good night, and had woken three times crying for a drink. She had not vomited once.

The following day she still had frequent diarrhoea, but was retaining fluids.

She made an uneventful recovery.

CASE 69

Emma, 10 months old

I was phoned for advice as Emma had had diarrhoea and vomiting for sixteen hours.

She was not retaining even water. *Phosphorus* had been ineffective, so I asked the parents to come to the surgery to collect *Aethusa* 200c granules, to be dissolved in half a cup of water, and to give half a teaspoon every half-hour. They were to phone the surgery in a couple of hours as I felt I would have to admit if there was no improvement.

Two hours later they phoned to say she was very much improved and had not vomited since the first dose.

Veratrum album (White Hellebore)

In toxic doses this plant powerfully affects the mind; the behaviour becomes either sullen or stuporous, or violent and destructive. It also produces gastritis, with a craving for cold water, which is vomited back immediately. In more serious cases there is profuse diarrhoea, with watery stools which are painfully and forcibly ejected. Severe calf cramps develop. Ultimately there is collapse, with icy coldness, cyanosis, and cold sweats, particularly of the forehead. All its discharges are copious: vomit, stools, urine, salivation and sweat.

With *Camphor* and *Cuprum*, *Veratrum album* was one of Hahnemann's three cholera medicines that so dramatically reduced the mortality rate when used in the cholera epidemics of his day. His successes were rewarded with hostility and bitter opposition from his colleagues, but he saved the lives of many people. His discovery of the curative power of these medicines also helped to establish homeopathy in the UK, because they were prescribed for cholera in 1854, in the London Homoeopathic Hospital, where the mortality figures were far less than those in all the other London hospitals.

The following two cases illustrate its use:

CASE 70
Kevin, age 14 years
This 14-year-old lad had had diarrhoea and vomiting for three days. He was now icy cold and covered with cold sweat. The parents had already tried *Phosphorus* and *Arsenicum album* from their home remedy kit, with no effect. He was given *Veratrum album* 10M dissolved in water, a teaspoonful every quarter of a hour, and an antiemetic suppository, and I asked for a report in two hours. Two hours later the parents reported that the suppository had not been necessary, that the vomiting had stopped very quickly and that their son was warm and sleeping soundly.

CASE 71
I was called to an urgent visit where the wife had fainted in the bathroom, having had relentless diarrhoea and vomiting all day.

Arsenicum album and *Phosphorus* had already been tried without effect. On examination on arrival, she was cold, with slight sweat on the forehead, and very weak. She was given *Veratrum album* 30c in water, a few sips to be taken every ten minutes. The husband was asked to telephone in the morning. *Veratrum* was chosen because of the severe prostration.

The following day I had heard nothing, so telephoned. The wife answered, 'Oh! I am sorry I had forgotten, I wasn't sick after the first sip and that medicine was the first fluid I was able to keep down all day.'

She was still weak, but the diarrhoea had stopped at the same time. She developed severe cramps during the night, and had I anticipated this I would have left her some *Cuprum* to follow.

By an interesting coincidence three of the five cases recorded were of events that took place at weekends. Our village pharmacy has always closed for the weekend at noon on Saturdays, and in those days the nearest chemist that was open for emergency out-of-hours dispensing was in Birmingham, over ten miles away. How convenient it has been for the patients that their GP has been able to carry over a hundred different homeopathic medicines, for emergency use, with him in his visiting case.

Podophyllum (May-apple)

CASE 72

A 2½-year-old boy had had teething diarrhoea for three weeks which had not responded to a kaolin mixture, which was the conventional treatment at the time.

The diarrhoea was always worse in the morning, and very malodorous – 'He smells the house out – like bad eggs.' His mother could not understand the 'terrific amount' of his stools, because he was not eating much. He was not ill in himself, nor miserable.

She had already tried *Arsenicum album* herself without benefit, so I gave him *Podophyllum* 12c, three doses to be taken that day, and subsequent doses as required.

She reported that she only needed to give three doses, as the diarrhoea stopped completely after the second dose.

Cocculus (Indian Cockle)

CASE 73

Stephen, a four-year-old boy, was always travel sick, and his father said he couldn't take him more than two miles by car at any time without him vomiting. I gave the father about a dozen pills of *Cocculus* 6c, one to be given fifteen minutes before the start of each journey.

He returned a few weeks later for a prescription for a further supply, and told me that they had worked on each occasion he had used them, but on the few occasions he had tried to leave them off 'there was trouble'.

As they appeared to be effective I increased the potency to 30c, which worked better, so that Stephen only took a dose at about weekly intervals. Within a few months he was able to discontinue the treatment.

Cocculus is included in the 'Homeopathic Travel Tablets', which also contain *Apomorphine*, *Theridion*, *Nux vomica*, *Petroleum*, *Staphysagria* and *Tabacum*.

These composite tablets are an example of homeopathic polypharmacy and are very useful, and can be bought from pharmacies and health shops without a prescription.

COLITIS

Secale cornutum (Ergot)

CASE 74

This history concerns a 60-year-old former night sister from Birmingham's largest teaching hospital, whom I had known thirty-five years previously when I was in residence as a newly qualified house physician.

She first consulted me on 23.4.77, when I failed to recognise her; she had lost weight, looked scrawny, gaunt, wasted and pale, and her voice had become husky and squeaky. Twelve years previously (1965) her husband had died suddenly and unexpectedly from a coronary thrombosis. A few months later she developed thyrotoxicosis, diagnosed by the professor of medicine, and was treated effectively with carbimazole 15 mg daily, which she had taken continuously since.

A year later (1966) she developed colitis, sufficient to incapacitate her and enforce early retirement from work. She had been prescribed an antidiarrhoeal tablet and now needed fourteen tablets daily to reduce the bowel frequency to four or five times daily. Her stools were bulky and malodorous. Her weight had fallen from 57 kg (125 lb) to 38 kg (84 lb) in the last year. She had a voracious appetite and intense thirst. Her throat was so dry she complained that it made it difficult for her to speak. She complained that her disposition had completely changed, that she was apathetic and irritable and easily upset. She was so exhausted she wanted to sit down all the time, or even stay in bed; her sister had to look after her. She could not tolerate a warm room. She suffered from intense paraesthesia 'like ants crawling all over me', particularly at night, so she wore silk gloves in bed to minimise the effects of scratching herself. She also suffered from 'dreadful calf cramps at night'. Despite all this she was very reluctant to consult her GP, who had not seen her for some time, but who had agreed to her telephone request that she should consult me for a homeopathic opinion.

She was 1.62 m tall (5 ft 4 in), normotensive (BP 120/80) and had no glycosuria.

Treatment

Continue conventional medication carbimazole 15 mg daily
An antidiarrhoeal (Lomotil) 14 tablets daily as required
Secale 200c, 3 doses on first day

I advised her to consult her GP with a view to seeing the professor of medicine again, or at least to having her thyroid function tests re-checked. I wrote to her GP informing him.

Her subsequent progress was as follows:

18.5.77. Very much improved – 'I feel so much better.'

Doing some housework, 'I cooked a meal for myself (first time for months).'

Bowel frequency reduced to twice daily, despite having gradually reduced the dose of Lomotil from fourteen a day until she had discontinued it altogether two days previously.

Attacks of formication reduced from several every night to one or two per week.

Gained 1.4 kg weight (3 lb) in the three weeks since taking *Secale* (first weight gain in the last two years).

Frequency and severity of calf cramps significantly decreased.

Has deferred consulting her GP and the professor of medicine!

Treatment

As I was concerned about whether she was still euthyroid, I changed her prescription:

Iodum 200c x 3 (three doses in one day)
Continue carbimazole 15 mg daily

I urged her to have her thyroid function tests checked.

17.8.77. No significant further improvement or weight gain.

Weight 39.5 kg (87 lb).

Feeling chilly, but was upset by the recent heatwave, and still cannot tolerate a warm room. Possibly a placebo would have been more appropriate than the *Iodum*, and I reverted to *Secale*.

Treatment

> *Secale* 200c x 3
> Carbimazole 15 mg daily

I insisted that she had her thyroid function retested.

She consulted the professor about two weeks later, who wrote (23.9.77): 'She has had a long history of thyrotoxicosis, the diagnosis of which seems correct in retrospect. She has not gained weight despite continuing carbimazole 5 mg, three times a day.

'She produces few symptoms of significance, but I found her to have a tremor, occasional extrasystoles, slightly warm palms and a diffuse hyperplastic thyroid gland. Clinically I thought she was probably euthyroid. The thyroid function tests have now come through and appear euthyroid although the serum triiodothyronine concentration is slightly on the high side. A complete blood count including ESR is normal. She has no glycosuria. It might be worth increasing her carbimazole slightly to 20 mg a day; if she does not improve in a month, I think we can assume her symptoms are not related to her thyroid gland.'

2.2.78. Dramatic improvement in appearance, weight and colour. Weight now 50.8 kg (112 lb).

Treatment

> No further homeopathic remedy at this point.
> Reduce carbimazole to 15 mg daily again

15.5.79. Now working again, helping disabled people. Feeling tired, and fearing a relapse of her earlier symptoms. Weight 51.3 kg (113 lb).

Treatment

> *Secale* 200c x 3
> Reduce carbimazole to 10 mg daily

23.9.80. She was doing a full day's work. Her weight was 52.5 kg (8 st 4 lb), her 'ideal weight'. She was only taking 5 mg carbimazole daily, and no other medication.

She reported she had 'had no formication or diarrhoea' from a month after her first attendance, despite having discontinued taking fourteen antidiarrhoeal tablets a day. This took place before she had temporarily increased the daily dose of carbimazole, as recommended by the professor of medicine.

I did not see her again, but her GP subsequently told me that she had maintained this improvement until she died a few years later from an unrelated cause.

Discussion

Various questions arise:

Was her dramatic improvement solely due to increasing her dose of carbimazole? Probably the weight gain between September 1977 and February 1978 was in response to a better control of her thyrotoxicosis, but her initial improvement between April and September 1977 occurred before her dose of carbimazole was changed. Could the formication have been iatrogenically induced? (Lomotil has been recorded as having produced allergic reactions, including urticaria and pruritus.) This was an unlikely cause because the regression of the formication preceded any significant reduction in the dose.

Was her excessive thirst, dry throat and husky voice due to the atropine in the Lomotil tablets? Probably, so those symptoms should not be used as reliable prescribing symptoms, though ergot poisoning produces them all.

Why was *Secale* chosen? The case was repertorised on the totality of symptoms that were most significant for homeopathic prescribing.

The most striking 'strange, rare and peculiar symptoms', therefore the most important for prescribing purposes, were:

Intense intolerance of external warmth – although she was emaciated, with no strength to move about to get warm and with minimal subcutaneous fat to keep her warm. Her formication was worse at night in bed and worse in a warm room.

Her skin felt cold, yet she neither felt the cold nor wanted warm clothing or bed clothing. At times she wanted to be uncovered. 'Skin cold, must uncover', *Camphor*, *Secale* only.

Gaunt scrawny appearance. 'Lean people', *Secale* (four bold type entries).

'Formication of skin' *Secale*
'Ravenous appetite' *Secale*
'Calf cramps' *Secale*
Note: Distinguish from 'Pain in calf'
'Indifference, apathy' *Secale*
'Weakness' *Secale*

Although weakness is a general symptom it is listed last, because I regarded it as a symptom common to the disease rather than a symptom of the patient. In other words, one would expect to find weakness as a result of her other debilitating symptoms, so the symptom of weakness is of little prescribing value.

If one eliminated the symptom 'Skin cold, must uncover' then four other medicines compete very closely with *Secale*. They are *Sulphur, Lycopodium, Phosphorus* and *Iodum*. They are all in each rubric either in bold type or italics, with the exception of 'warm' in *Phosphorus*, and 'apathy' and 'formication' in *Iodum*, all of which are in small type.

Summary

Secale would appear to have initially helped her lassitude, diarrhoea, formication, calf cramps and above all, her apathy, restoring to her a sense of wellbeing. The further marked improvement that followed the therapeutic trial of increasing her dose of carbimazole suggests that she was still slightly thyrotoxic, and the indicated homeopathic medicine was not sufficient on its own. This case illustrates that homeopathic medicines can be of benefit when taken concurrently with conventional drugs.

CROHN'S DISEASE

In my experience patients consult a homeopathic doctor in desperation because they have failed to respond to current conventional treatment. It is not simply a matter of 'I don't want to take drugs' – they will take anything that alleviates their symptoms.

The first point I emphasise to my patients, and mention in my letter to their GP, is that homeopathy will, in their case, only be an additional form of therapy. The patient should continue taking whatever conventional medication the GP or consultant involved feels is indicated. This is mandatory if the patient is taking maintenance steroids, as it is imperative that they do not suddenly discontinue taking them when they have been on them for years, or even only months.

Aims of Homeopathic Treatment in Crohn's Disease

- An improvement in the patient's sense of wellbeing and outlook.
- A steady decrease in the severity of their symptoms, of pain, wind and cramps, and a reduction of the number of times they have their bowels open.
- The ability to resume eating a full diet, and regain the weight lost on account of their illness.
- That they may be able to reduce, and possibly ultimately discontinue, the dose of corticosteroids.
- That the patient can reduce analgesics and antidiarrhoea drugs.
- To provide specific therapy for surgical complications, possibly aborting abscess formation, accelerating the healing of fistulae and perianal inflammatory lesions, and prevent the need for further resections.

Where appropriate I advise on modifying the patient's lifestyle, on reducing stress, and on diet. I also discuss their smoking habits, though in the series presented below, only one acted on my advice on smoking.

Homeopathic Prescribing Symptoms

As in all homeopathic prescribing, one must look for unusual symptoms peculiar to the patient, tending to discard symptoms common to the disease. We also have to ignore symptoms produced by the conventional medication that is currently being taken. Unless one has complete responsibility for the patient, it would be unethical and irresponsible to instruct them to discontinue conventional treatment so that we could start again with an uncomplicated picture of their symptoms. Consequently, some symptoms, such as thirst, dry mouth, nausea, etc., may have to be ignored. I tend to discount them unless they are strikingly prominent.

Prescribing

When I can identify the patient's constitutional medicine (and often it is not clear-cut) or the medicine that covers the totality of symptoms, I prescribe it in a 30c or 200c potency, to be repeated according to the patient's response, at intervals of three to fourteen days. I also prescribe a 'local' medicine that specifically matches the bowel symptoms, to be taken frequently in low potency on the intervening days (i.e. 3c–6c, every hour to two hours). My reason for this is that in private practice patients come long distances, often with difficulty, and unless very well motivated towards homeopathic treatment will not re-attend and pay a second consultation fee unless they obtained significant improvement following their first visit. Hence the use of a local medicine which should predictably alleviate some symptoms, and possibly lessen the severity of any aggravation, should it occur.

I also use the following nosodes:

- *Proteus*, if there has been prolonged nervous strain, or cramps.
- *Dysenteriae co.*, where nervous tension or anticipatory fears are prominent.
- *Gaertner*, where there is marked weight loss and malnutrition, and where *Phosphorus* has proved very effective.
- *Tuberculinum* because of the similarity between Crohn's disease and tuberculosis, which often confuses the diagnosis, and because *Mycobacterium paratuberculosis*, an organism which causes a granulomatous intestinal inflammation (Johne's disease) in farm animals, has been isolated from a few patients with Crohn's disease.
- A nosode of *E. coli* using, if obtainable, a preparation made from the enteroadherent serotype of the diarrhoeagenic strain (isopathy).

Study

In a series of sixteen patients (Jack, R.A.F. 'How I treat Crohn's disease.' *British Homoeopathic Journal*, 1993; 82: 29–36), eleven were female and ten were smokers.

The constitutional medicines which apparently were most effective were, in order of frequency, and number of cases:

Phosphorus 7
Phosphoric acid 6
Nux vomica 4
Lycopodium 2
Pulsatilla 1

The most effective 'local' medicines were:

Podophyllum (10)
Aloe (6)

Some patients required, and responded to, two different constitutional medicines during their course of treatment.

Comments

Both *Phosphorus* and *Phosphoric acid* produce debilitating painless diarrhoea – hence their usefulness in cases of Crohn's disease where pain associated with defaecation is minimal. Interestingly, Hahnemann only proved *Phosphorus* some time after he had published the provings of *Phosphoric acid* in his *Materia Medica Pura*. Already over seventy years old, and living in Paris, he was mainly treating chronic illnesses, which frequently did not respond to the medicines he had available. He began to formulate his theory of chronic disease, and tested fifteen extra medicines, including *Phosphorus*, to meet his need.

Prescribing indications for local medicines:

- *Podophyllum* is indicated for profuse morning diarrhoea when the stool is particularly malodorous. A useful aide-memoire is: Profuse Offensive Dawn
- *Aloe* is effective for abdominal distension with rectal insecurity – unsure whether flatus or faeces will be passed. ('I daren't pass wind.')
- *Gambogia* has similar distension, but more borborygmi, more tenesmus, and the stool is more forcibly and suddenly ejected.

CASE 75

Female, 56 years old, 23-year history of Crohn's, referred by her GP.

She had had four bowel resections (1955, 1962, 1971 and 1973). First attended 26.4.78. 'Professor of surgery told me that there was very little large intestine left, and much of small bowel had been removed and that each operation shortens the gut and makes recovery less likely.' Multiple allergies to antibiotics. Had severe reaction to tetracycline which produced cramps, severe diarrhoea and vomiting leading to collapse, unconsciousness and admission to hospital, requiring intravenous infusion, and in-patient treatment for one month. Still attending hospital monthly. Her medication was folic acid, multivitamins and injections of vitamin B12. She complained of:

Painless urgent diarrhoea, bowels opened five to ten times daily (occasionally twenty times). Watery, foamy, only occasionally formed stool. No blood. No rectal incontinence but she 'daren't pass wind'. Burning in stomach after eating anything, only relieved by ice-cold milk. Insatiable thirst. Drinks pints until bloated, but 'it doesn't quench my thirst.'

Prescribing features:

Chilly, intolerant of the cold, and feels cold internally (except stomach).

Needs hot water bottles.

Gets feverish attacks and rigors.

Very weak and exhausted. 'Thunder headaches', vertigo, spontaneous bruises.

As a person she was artistic, sympathetic, 'moved by sunset, and music'. Hypersensitive to sound.

She had no irrational fears but otherwise was a typical *Phosphorus* type.

Treatment

26.4.78. *Phosphorus* 30c, then 200c three days later. *Podophyllum* 12c every two hours in attacks of diarrhoea.

As she lived 125 miles away across country, most consultations that followed were by telephone.

10.5.78. '*Podophyllum* marvellous. Makes the stool slightly formed after three hours.'

Treatment

Podophyllum 30c as required.

30.5.78. '*Podophyllum* 30c works better than 12c. No diarrhoea for two days – unprecedented in twenty years. Thrilled.'

27.8.78. Urgent phone call, 'No bowel movement for 21 hours – is that all right?'!

Developing very severe cramps and spasms of body and limbs.

Treatment

Cuprum 30c three times a day.

She later wrote to report that *Cuprum* was very effective.

During 1979 she found *China* 30c eased her episodes of abdominal distension, *Phosphoric acid* 12c helped her lassitude, and she had *Morgan Gaertner* 30c (single dose).

By 1980 bowels opened three to five times daily. She had resumed all social activities which had been abandoned in the decade before taking homeopathic medicines. She was still taking her conventional medication and using homeopathic medicines as well, when required. In the next eleven years I saw her twice (1983) and she phoned me ten times.

In 1983 she developed an ischiorectal abscess which did not heal. 'The pus soaked the dressings four times daily' until she took *Hepar sulph.* 6c four times a day, followed by *Silica* 10M two days later. 'The effect was dramatic.'

1984. Similar episode and response.

24.1.92. Phoned. Relapse of rectal abscesses, and diarrhoea, uncontrolled by *Podophyllum*. Finds *Carbo veg.* helps her wind. Bowels opened eight times daily.

Treatment

Aloe 6c four times a day for diarrhoea.
Gambogia 6c four times a day if *Aloe* does not work.

5.2.92. Diarrhoea did not respond to *Aloe*, but *Gambogia* worked well.

17.6.92. Attended with recurrence of rectal abscesses and diarrhoea.

Treatment

Tuberculinum 10M x 1 (see page 131), and a week later start *E. coli* 30c one dose a day for seven days, reducing to one dose a week thereafter.

Discussion

Although not enjoying good health at the age of 70 years (with angina and circulatory problems), her health in the fourteen years since she had had homeopathic treatment was far better than in the previous twenty-three years, during which time she had had four resections and four operations on account of abscesses. She attributed this improvement to homeopathy, and I confess I had to agree with her!

CASE 76

Female, aged 24 years, diagnosed as suffering from Crohn's disease six years before she first saw me on 3.9.84.

She was still under a gastroenterologist who had fully investigated her. She was 1.63 m (5 ft 4 in) tall and weighed 54 kg (119 lb) and she smoked five to ten cigarettes daily. Although taking a high roughage diet she found it had not significantly helped. She complained of diarrhoea and recurrent abdominal pain.

Despite taking sulphasalazine 500 mg eight times a day for the previous five years continuously, she still had her bowels open ten to eighteen times a day, predictably more frequently in the morning. The stools were bulky and malodorous.

She was a chilly woman who liked warm rooms, loved heatwaves and sunbathing. She wanted company, bruised easily, was thirsty and liked salty foods.

Treatment

3.9.84. *Phosphorus* 30c one a week (single dose).
Podophyllum 3c four times a day.
Continue sulphasalazine eight per day.

I also suggested she tried a wheat exclusion diet for five days and gave her instructions concerning her cigarette smoking.
1.10.84. 'Feeling very much improved, 50% better.' Bowels opened only five to eight times a day, and stool more formed and less fluid. No change on wheat-free diet.
'After each dose of *Phosphorus* I improve noticeably for the next twenty-four hours.'

Treatment

Phosphorus 30c alternate mornings, reducing to every third or fourth morning with improvement.
Podophyllum 3c four times a day.
Continue sulphasalazine eight times a day.

26.11.84. Still feeling 50% improved (husband agrees).
Bowels open still five to eight times daily, though a change in bowel habit. Diarrhoea no longer mornings, but 'Immediate urge after a mouthful of food, or any hot drink. Must have bowels open within a minute, or possibly an accident.' Feels need of *Phosphorus* every forty-eight hours.

Treatment

Phosphorus 30c every second day.
Replace *Podophyllum* with *Aloe* 3c four times a day.
Sulphasalazine eight times a day – suggest asking her GP if she could try gradually reducing this dose.

11.2.85. Without reference to her GP she stopped sulphasalazine completely the day following her last consultation, apparently without any untoward reaction: 'I haven't missed them at all.' Bowels open five to six times daily, twice in the morning before work, three or four times in the afternoon after work. Diarrhoea no longer urgent after food. Abdominal pain now minimal, only before urge to stool and eased after defaecation. 'I now dare to go to places where there may not be a toilet.'

Treatment

Phosphorus 10M x 1.
Resume *Phosphorus* 30c after a week, if required, at two to three day intervals. *Aloe* 3c three times a day.

13.5.85. Relapsing, 'not feeling so good'.

Treatment

Tub. bov. 10M x 1 (possible link between Johne's tubercular bowel disease in cattle, and Crohn's disease).

17.6.85. 'Very much improved after *Tub. bov.* – 60% improvement.' Bowels open two or three times in the morning and two or three times in the afternoon.

Treatment

Continue *Phosphorus* 30c and *Aloe* 3c as before.

1.10.85. 'Now 65% improved.' Bowels open twice before 9 a.m. and occasionally not at all in the evening. Asking for a second dose of *Tub. bov.* Attending fertility clinic.

Treatment

Tub. bov. 10M x 1.
Phosphorus 30c three times a week.
Trial *Podophyllum* 200c in two weeks time.

11.2.86. Letter cancelling her appointment '... because I felt so well ..., I am expecting a baby in May, and being pregnant has seemed to help my complaint, but I cannot thank you enough for helping me to get better. Some days I do not need to go to the toilet at all, which is quite different from a year ago. I am still taking the tablets you prescribed.'

Discussion

June 1992. Sad sequel. I telephoned her for information about her subsequent progress. Apparently she had enjoyed two years of 'feeling fine', followed by a traumatic divorce, and the death of her mother. She then had an ovarian cyst removed and states that she was told in hospital that her relapse was 'due to homeopathy' (her consultant had previously upset her by his antagonism to homeopathy, so she had ceased attending him). Whatever was told her had the effect of making her stop taking homeopathic medicines altogether. She deteriorated, was referred to a professor of surgery, and this year had a colectomy and an ileostomy. She now is not taking any homeopathic medicines, yet is not being prescribed any conventional treatment! She has remarried, and is 'managing well' with her ileostomy.

CASE 77

A young man 19 years old, whose mother is Austrian, first consulted me for Crohn's disease on 22.2.88.

Two years previously, when on holiday in Austria, he had an emergency appendicectomy, was flown home, and was admitted to an English hospital on account of increasing colic. Crohn's disease was diagnosed and an ileostomy performed. His condition deteriorated, and he was warned he would probably need a colectomy; hence his interest in an alternative therapy. He hoped homeopathic treatment would not only spare him needing a resection, but also so improve his health that he could have his ileostomy reversed.

He had been unemployed for two years, chiefly because of this illness. He had lost 6.3 kg (14 lb) in weight, and was now 57 kg (126 lb), and 1.75 m (5 ft 9 in) tall.

He smoked approximately ten cigarettes daily.

He had discontinued taking sulphasalazine, and used two prednisolone suppositories twice a day.

His presenting symptoms were extreme lassitude, and perianal discomfort because of inflammation from infections, resulting in an intermittent bloodstained rectal discharge.

His significant prescribing features were:

Profound lassitude, listless and apathetic in appearance, pallor.

Long-continued painless diarrhoea, stools not offensive.

He was chilly and loved heatwaves.

Craving for salt and three pints of cold milk daily.

Treatment

22.2.88. *Phosphoric acid* 10M x 1. Experimentally, I added *Phosphoric acid* 6c three times a day. Continue prednisolone suppositories twice a day. Instructions about reducing smoking.

20.3.88. '60% improved, less exhausted.' Rectal infection subsiding.

Treatment

Phosphorus 10M x 1.
Phosphoric acid 6c two to three times a day.
Prednisolone suppositories twice daily.

29.4.88. '90% improvement.' Feeling much better, 'confident they will be able to close my ileostomy.' 'Feel like job hunting again; I could work a full day. Rectum less sore – discharge much less. I no longer crave milk, and have halved the amount I drink.'

Treatment

Phosphorus 1M x 1.
Phosphoric acid 6c twice a day.
Prednisolone suppositories as required.

30.1.89. Returned from abroad, where he had worked in a German hotel for four months and enjoyed it. He had stopped all medication, although he still smoked as much as before. Still slight rectal discharge. Feeling well.

Intending returning to Germany to work in a better hotel.

June 1992. Unable to contact him.

CASE 78

Mr. S.A., age 26 years, first attended me for homeopathic treatment on 3.9.90.

His doctor's letter stated: 'He has suffered from Crohn's disease since 1984. A recent barium meal and follow-through showed multiple strictures in his ileum, and I recently admitted him to hospital with subacute obstruction. He is on prednisolone 25 mg daily.' He had been on prednisolone for six years, initially on a smaller dose, but inexorably he had to increase it over the years, relapsing every time he cautiously tried reducing the dose. He had also taken sulphasalazine, but discontinued it as it had not helped in any way.

He was a bachelor, 1.87 m (6 ft 1 in) tall, and weighed 66.7 kg (147 lb); he had never smoked and had been a keen cyclist and badminton player till his illness had incapacitated him. He complained of recurrent attacks of bloating, 'burning indigestion', both partially relieved by belching or passing flatus. The attacks lasted six or seven hours and were followed by a 'strange optimistic feeling'. Prednisolone 20 mg enemas had been helpful in the past, but now were ineffective. His diarrhoea was controlled with treatment; he only had one or two bowel actions daily.

His problem was that his condition made him feel exhausted, impatient and irritable. He said he was 'a shy loner', and on questioning admitted he was a 'conscientious worrier'. He stated he was 'fanatically tidy', liked sympathy, was quick and decisive, but not competitive.

He was stubborn and could speak his mind. He was warm-blooded, liked windows open and fresh air, and bruised easily. He was not a thirsty person, had never liked salty foods, nor had he a craving for sweets.

I considered and eliminated *Nux vomica*, *Phosphorus* and even *Arsenicum album* as his constitutional medicine; his symptoms on balance pointed to *Lycopodium*, even though he did not have a pronounced 4–8 p.m. aggravation, nor a craving for sweets. As a minor confirmatory clue I noted that he was always frowning.

Treatment

3.9.90. *Lycopodium* 30c twice a day until reaction (i.e. getting better or worse, then withhold the medicine until it ceased acting).
Continue prednisolone 25 mg daily, unless his GP decided to alter the dose.

1.10.90. 'Improvement 30%. Not feeling so worried about my condition. No bloating at all – most surprised as unprecedented. Stomach pains have altered and are preceded by increased impatience and irritability. My consultant has been able to reduce my steroids to 20 mg prednisolone daily.'

Treatment

Lycopodium 10M x 1.
7 days later, if required, resume *Lycopodium* 30c twice a day at two to seven day intervals, according to response.
Nux vomica 30c four times a day for colic and excessive irritability.
Prednisolone 20 mg daily.

5.11.90. '65% improved. Virtually pain-free last five weeks. No bloating, no burning. I have resumed cycling and playing badminton.'
11.2.91. 'Fine, until I tried reducing prednisolone below 17.5 mg daily.'
Relapse of abdominal pain.

Treatment

Add *Colocynthis* 30c as required when attacks of colic better for pressure, better for warm applications, better for doubling up. To try *Magnesia phosphorica* 30c if no response to *Colocynthis*.

11.3.91. '80% better. Only two mild episodes of burning abdominal pain in last month.' Prednisolone down to 16 mg daily for last two weeks.

29.4.91. Increase in attacks of colic. No response to *Colocynthis*; improved on *Mag. phos.* (Problem with next-door neighbour who is planning to build an extension which will effectively block out his light, etc.)

Treatment

Proteus 10M x 1. Prednisolone now 14 mg daily.

26.6.91. 'Fine, no problems. Close on 100% fit.' Reduced prednisolone to 13 mg daily. 'I always notice lassitude the day I reduce the prednisolone and the following day.' Is on course of iron tablets for his anaemia.

Treatment

Lycopodium 10M x 1.
Lycopodium 30c when necessary.
Prednisolone now 12.5 mg daily.

30.9.91. 'Feeling well on 12.5 mg prednisolone for the last two weeks. An unprecedented low dose for me.' Return of mild episodes of 'burning and bloating' every seven to ten days. Still cycling and playing badminton. Main concern today is relapse of his facial acne.

Treatment:

Natrum bromatum 200c x 1 (for his acne).
Carbo veg. 30c trial instead of *Mag phos.*
Continue *Lycopodium* 30c as required.
Prednisolone 12.5 mg daily.

24.2.92. Maintaining improvement and quality of life.
Recent holiday in Australia for two months. Prednisolone 12.5 mg daily (was 25 mg for last few years).
30.6.92. Maintaining improvement.

BUCCAL ULCERS

CASE 79

A 59-year-old successful quantity surveyor had suffered from recurrent crops of bilateral painful buccal ulcers for over forty years. They were so painful that he had got into the habit of speaking through his teeth, without moving his jaws. He was lucky if he got four or five days freedom between the attacks, and the ulcers were so sensitive that while they lasted he could only eat sloppy foods like bread and milk. In one very severe attack he could not eat properly for three months, and lost 4kg (9lb) in weight.

He was seen by a consultant, who diagnosed a viral infection but offered no treatment. Indeed, none of the accepted treatments gave him any relief, except hydrocortisone pellets, which he used four times a day. Finally he developed a prolonged viral throat infection followed by the post-viral fatigue syndrome, and after he had been off work for three months, in desperation he turned to homeopathy as his last hope.

My immediate reaction to his story was that he must have a masked food intolerance, i.e. an allergy to a food he craved for and ate regularly. His wife, who accompanied him, confirmed his story, and listed the foods they had positively identified, or which aggravated his ulcers. She said, 'He can tell at once when he has eaten the wrong thing, as his mouth smarts immediately.' He was a neat, active and dapper man who now felt very weak, chilly and restless, both mentally and physically. He enjoyed eating animal fat, which he could tolerate; he found it 'tasty'. Checking the rubric in Kent's *Repertory* for mouth ulcers, the prominent black letter drugs listed are: ARS. ALB., IOD., KALI IOD., LACH., MERC., MUR. AC, NIT. AC.

Arsenicum album was the medicine that best matched his symptoms.

I prescribed *Arsenicum album* 30c two a day, every fourth day, as his condition was urgent, rather than waiting to test an exclusion diet before treatment. He returned four weeks later, stating, 'I am 90% better. I haven't had a single ulcer since the first dose, although several times my mouth has started smarting, as if an attack was imminent, but each time it aborted. I have been eating things I never dared to try previously.' He had only used one hydrocortisone pellet in the last three weeks. 'I am very pleased after all the years I have suffered.' I reduced his dose of *Arsenicum album* 30c to two a day, every fifth day.

A month later he claimed 100% success, not a single symptom in the preceding two weeks.

141

He was now eating all the foods that had formerly been proscribed. His wife commented on how 'the ulcers in the past had totally affected his health and work input'. A month later I presented him and his wife at the 51st Tutorial of the Midlands Branch of the Faculty of Homeopathy. He was still taking occasional doses of *Arsenicum album* 30c for fear of relapsing. He mentioned then for the first time that he had had a longstanding anal irritation, but that it had been alleviated since taking *Arsenicum album.*

Chapter 10

Female Reproductive System

Gynaecological problems are very common in general practice, and homeopathy can be of great help with conditions that are difficult to treat conventionally, such as premenstrual tension.

PREMENSTRUAL TENSION (PMT)

CASE 80

A 37-year-old beauty consultant had suffered from severe PMT for six years, during which time she had had private treatment by a leading Birmingham gynaecologist. Diuretics, tranquillisers, pyridoxine (Vitamin B6) and danazol had not controlled her symptoms, and progesterone suppositories inserted at four-hour intervals only gave some relief, but had to be discontinued as she became allergic to them.

Her menstrual cycle length had always been twenty-one to twenty-eight days, but for the last three months had come every three weeks. Her periods were moderate, and she had neither dysmenorrhoea or dyspareunia (pain on intercourse). She had only minimal fluid retention and weight gain. Her breasts became tender, but she did not develop a headache, nor become accident prone.

Her problem was: 'Two weeks premenstrually I develop a complete personality change. Everybody is wrong, no one can please me. I become totally unpredictable, with verbal nastiness mainly towards my family, but also to clients and others. I fly off the handle at nothing. I fall out with myself, even when alone in the house. I become nasty and violent to my kids (two girls), and could lash out at them and be very, very nasty to my husband. I have to mark off the days in my diary and stay at home, and I just have to go through it.'

I asked her about her attitude to sex. 'In the premenstrual week I am well, I am an affectionate person and still like a cuddle – but no more. No, I'm not hostile to sex.'

I gave her a single dose of *Natrum mur.* 10M, to be repeated every fifteenth day of her cycle, and a prescription for *Nux vomica* 10M to be

143

taken at the onset of her vicious moods, and repeated every one to two hours as required.

I questioned her about the relationship between her mental symptoms and the onset of her periods. Until three months ago she was 'regular to the hour. The minute my period starts everything lifts. I know I've started even before I feel damp down below'.

She returned two months later – exuberant. Her periods had reverted to a four-week cycle, and her PMT was markedly improved. Each morning, the moment she felt nasty she took *Nux vomica* 10M and usually only had to take one or two more doses during the morning. The benefit seemed to last through the next day. 'Will I have to take these for the rest of my life?' I explained that homeopathic medicines alleviated conditions by curing, rather than suppressing the symptoms, which tend to become progressively less severe, less frequent and less in duration.

This is what happened in her case. At her third visit two months later she used the words 'super' and 'marvellous'. She had 'only had three bad days' since she last attended and they were nothing like as bad as they had been. 'I'm a different person now, and my husband agrees. My stomach has settled, I don't get the tension in it any longer.'

She did have to take both medicines intermittently for the next year.

Kent in his repertory lists medicines which treat conditions which are either aggravated or ameliorated by the menses.

For PMT that resolves immediately the flow starts, the most prominent medicines are *Calc. carb.*, *Natrum mur.*, *Lachesis*, *Pulsatilla*, *Sepia* and *Sulphur*. *Nux vomica* is included, but only in small print, as it is listed in large bold type among the medicines indicated when the symptoms are aggravated during or after the menses. A typical example would be a woman whose periods were too frequent and heavy, with dysmenorrhoea and menorrhagia, associated with nausea and/or sickness, and with ineffectual bowel actions, and irritability.

In this case the mental symptoms were so dominant, and so typical of *Nux*, that I prescribed it in high potency. Later I gave her a few doses of *Nux* CM to try, but she found that she could not detect any greater benefit than when using the 10M potency.

It is a pity that the Greek philosopher who wrote: 'There is a time in the month when every woman should live at the bottom of the garden' had not tried giving *Nux* in potency to his unfortunate wife!

CASE 81

She was twenty-four years old, with a 4-year-old son, whom she referred to as 'Bab'. I had been her doctor since childhood.

She complained of the side effects of her contraceptive pill. The recording of her uninhibited account of her complaints, in the local vernacular and dialect is fascinating to listen to:

'Do you think it might be the Pill? When I come off them it's terrible, lethal. I've had no period for twelve months, just a little discharge for one day. When I'm off them I'm a misery; they will tell you at work. I keep crying, I don't know what for. I'm OK on the Pill – puts me on Cloud 9, but I am getting fatter and fatter.' She had been on a high-oestrogen oral contraceptive pill for years but after gaining 22.7 kg (50 lb) the family planning clinic prescribed a lower oestrogen substitute.

'I get false alarms with my bowels, and I become vile. I could strangle Bab and kill him. He says "Me mum's got miseries". I feel the cold, shuts the windows and puts the heating on to 27°C (80°F). I'm always froze. No, I don't get flushes or sweats – wish I did to get hotted up.'

'For the first day off the Pill I get a headache and go mad. I get a terrible temper. I'm vile, murderous. I throw things about – smash cups on the wall – two a day, and ruin the wallpaper. Yes, I fly off the handle. I'm so bad my mum tape-recorded me so I could listen to it. I'm driving my husband mad. He says I'm a head-case. He used to work in a mental hospital. I'm going barmy, crazy – yet afterwards I can laugh at it.'

I prescribed *Nux vomica* 30c, telling her to use her own supply which she had among her home remedy set, and which she had used for 'Bab' when he was constipated, but had never taken herself.

She returned after her next period – a very grateful woman. The *Nux* appeared to have controlled her temper tantrums and headache, and restored calm in the home.

In the following fifteen years she has resorted to *Nux* from time to time, which has effectively prevented or controlled recurrences of her premenstrual outbursts of aggression and violence.

When a mother suffers from severe PMT of this sort, and has a fractious teething baby, the stage is set for a battered baby. In my opinion the tragedy could be averted in many cases if the mother took *Nux*, and gave the babe *Chamomilla*.

CASE 82

A 33-year-old woman complained of premenstrual fluid retention; total lack of energy and depression. She was 30% overweight, and in the week before her periods gained another 2.7 kg (6 lb). She stopped weighing herself as it only made her more despondent, and started measuring herself instead. She gained between one and two inches around her bust and waist. At times she felt 'almost suicidal'.

She became intolerant of a hot room and tight clothing. Her nadir of mood was always in the morning, and her mental symptoms resolved immediately she started menstruating.

So far the most useful prescribing clues were:

- Depression before periods.
- Aggravation after sleep.
- Fluid retention (in Kent under 'Generalities', sub-section 'swelling, puffy').
- Worse for warmth.

Computer analysis reveals that among the many medicines that are indicated for that cluster of symptoms, *Lycopodium*, *Sepia*, *Lachesis*, *Calcarea* and *Pulsatilla* head the list in that order, but with very little to choose between them.

I then asked more personal questions which I usually leave until later in an interview, unless I know the patient well, and I elucidated that during the pre-menstrual phase she became more talkative than usual and rather suspicious.

'Strange you ask that. Yes, I do. I know its ridiculous but if my husband is quarter of an hour late coming home, I automatically feel he is having an affair with another woman.'

'Does your PMT make you feel jealous?' 'Yes' she said, 'if I come into the room, and see him enjoying watching a glamorous blonde on TV or a scantily dressed woman dancing I become so upset I have to leave the room.'

Adding in these unusual mental changes gave *Lachesis* a clear lead over the other medicines, and the extra facts I then elicited – that she preferred the autumn to spring and summer, and that her face often went slightly purplish, confirmed my choices.

I gave her three doses of *Lachesis* 200c, one to be taken monthly at the onset of her PMT, and three months later she returned for a prescription. She was delighted and most grateful for her improvement. Her depression and PMT had been completely controlled, and she could 'now look back and laugh at her jealousies and suspicions'.

CASE 83

A 38-year-old woman complained about her irritability and depression. She could not stand the noise of the children and wanted to get away, or be left alone at home. Her libido was flat; she had an antagonism to sex, and felt there was a 'lump in her vagina'. She was always hungry, but eating did not satiate her.

Although she was 'overjoyed' when the house was empty, she became obsessed with unreasonable fears as to what was happening to her husband, children or father when they were out of her presence. When she was upset she got angry with anyone who tried to console her.

She developed an intolerance to tobacco smoke, and her hair kept coming out in combfuls, despite having a course of massage from her hairdresser.

She began to hate herself for feeling like this: it was 'so out of character'.

On these strong mental changes I prescribed a single dose of *Sepia* 200c and gave her three spare doses to take at intervals of 7–28 days according to her response.

When she returned three months later she was delighted with her treatment, and in recounting her improvement added new details of her previous symptoms and problems.

Her depression had lifted: 'I had forgotten what the trees and sky looked like'; her hair stopped falling out; she had lost her irritability: 'I didn't want anyone about – not the kids or the cat or the dog. If anyone cried "Mummy" I'd scream. Now if they said "Mummy" six times, I'd smile. My sex drive has returned. My husband says it is the best in fifteen years of marriage: it is the first time he couldn't cope with me. He was going to send you a telegram, it is absolutely marvellous. My palpitations and PMT have virtually disappeared. My periods, which had been every three weeks, have reverted to every four weeks.'

All this improvement was starting to wear off so I gave her a prescription for *Sepia* 200c which she took at infrequent intervals, which controlled her symptoms for the next six years, when I lost touch with her.

Prescribing Analysis

For prescribing the indicated remedy, the most significant strong mental and physical complaints are listed, with the appropriate rubric and page number in Kent's *Repertory*. Also, the number of medicines

147

in that rubric is included, and the rank of *Sepia* in each case is shown (3 = heavy black type, 2 = italics).

Rubric	Kent page	No. of remedies	Rank
Anxiety with fear	6	80	3
Aversion to coition	715	47	3
Aversion to company	12	100	2
Ball internally	1345	36	3
Emptiness not relieved by eating	488	40	3
Head; hair falling	120	120	3
Indifference to loved ones	55	9	3
Prostration of mind	70	77	3

One long-suffering husband once complained 'Putting my arms round my wife is like putting them round the office cabinet!' He took some *Sepia* 200c for her, and they were both so delighted with the result that they became enthusiastic supporters of homeopathy. In my experience, *Sepia* has been the most indicated remedy for those who have become loveless towards their kith and kin, and are distressed about it.

MITTELSCHMERZ

CASE 84

A 43-year-old woman had suffered from 'Mittelschmerz' (mid-cycle pain) for four years, which had not been controlled by strong analgesics or fenoprofen. She also suffered from ten days of premenstrual mastalgia, and on my direct questioning, to confirm the remedy choice, she admitted that she had rheumatic pains in both her thumbs.

I gave her a single dose of *Cimicifuga* 1M and a prescription for *Cimicifuga* 3c four times a day for her ovulatory pain. This prescription was based on the predilection of *Cimicifuga* for the ovary and also for the small joints of the hand.

Three months later she reported that for the first month on this treatment her pain was 90% relieved, and for the following two months both her abdominal colic and her breast pains had completely disappeared. Her menstrual cycle had extended from twenty-four days, which had been her pattern for many years, to twenty-six days.

She asked 'How does that medicine work – is it all in the mind?' Added to this her arthritic thumbs had been completely pain-free after the first month. In the past she could bring on the pain simply by putting her hands in cold water, but not now. I explained how she should try reducing her medication, and as far as I am aware the treatment remained effective until her menopause, when her problems resolved.

MENORRHAGIA

CASE 85

A 34-year-old woman had suffered from menorrhagia for five years, despite treatment at the Women's Hospital during that time. Her periods lasted for seven days, and the cycle length was twenty days. As she was seeking further help and her full investigations had eliminated sinister pathology, I decided to try homeopathy.

She was a typical *Natrum mur.* type. She confessed to being a somewhat self-willed, irritable person, who resented consolation when upset. She did not like the heat and could not sunbathe. She loved salty foods, and was thirsty.

I gave her *Natrum mur.* 30c, three doses in one day.

When she next attended, she said: 'I couldn't believe it. Eighteen months ago you gave me three pills for my flooding which I'd had for five years, and my periods became normal again.' In the last three months her symptoms were returning, and she had recently developed cystitis, with terminal dysuria. I prescribed *Sarsaparilla* 3c alternate hours, and arranged for a midstream urine analysis, which was negative. She found *Sarsaparilla* very effective, and when her cystitis settled she was given *Natrum mur.* 200c, following which her menorrhagia subsided again.

BREAST PROBLEMS

CASE 86

A 44-year-old woman suddenly developed mastalgia, with very severe pain in her nipple. It started as a burning pain but quickly changed to a 'sticking pain which got worse and worse and worse'. It was 'a terrible pain, real agony'. There had been a slight milky discharge, which was unprecedented. Since her periods had always been irregular she was unable to say she was now premenstrual. The breasts were not hot, either objectively or subjectively and there was no deep tenderness, but the ends of both nipples were swollen and very red.

She had attended one of my partners four days previously who had prescribed co-proxamol, and reasonably suggested she tried first

Belladonna 30c, and if that failed to relieve, *Phosphorus* 30c. The pain persisted, and in fact was getting worse.

I saw her in morning surgery. She looked washed out and tearful; she had not slept for the last four nights because of the pain. I asked her if the pain was like nettle stings. 'Yes, but much much worse.' I gave her a supply of *Urtica urens* 12c, one to be taken every alternate hour until improvement, and a prescription for more should she find them effective and need more.

She returned by appointment the next morning. The pain had eased significantly by lunch time the previous day, and was bearable. She had had a good night's sleep and the pain had subsided. To my knowledge the condition has not recurred in the following nineteen years. (Needless to say, if the symptoms had not quickly settled, I would have referred her to exclude carcinoma.)

CASE 87

Gwendoline, aged 45, complained of heaviness in the breasts and tender, sore nipples from the fourteenth to twenty-eighth day of each menstrual cycle, for the last twelve years. Worse for jarring, worse walking down stairs. Symptoms worse in the last four months.

On these symptoms, I prescribed *Phytolacca* 12c, three times a day until relief.

Three months later, she reported that her symptoms were very much improved. The pain and nipple tenderness now occurred only on the 24th–28th days of the cycle.

I gave her *Phytolacca* CM, on alternate days until relief, starting on the twentieth day of the cycle.

Four months later she reported that she was 'Marvellous. I take one pill when the discomfort starts seven days before my period and occasionally need a second dose a few days afterwards.'

CASE 88

A 26-year-old woman, two weeks post-partum, awake all night with her breast throbbing and burning.

On examining her, there was an inflammatory reaction around the nipple, which was hot to touch – 'burning and throbbing'.

I gave *Belladonna* 200c in water, to be sipped at frequent intervals. I also gave a prescription for antibiotics to take if the pain had not subsided by the morning.

The next day, all the heat and redness had gone, and she was delighted, and had not needed or taken any antibiotics.

PRURITUS VULVAE

CASE 89

A 35-year-old nurse suffered from distressing pruritus vulvae. She said the irritation was 'distressing, you can't really describe it, it is un-bearable. Cortisone cream makes no difference.' I prescribed tincture of nettle (*Urtica urens*), ten drops to be diluted in half a cup of cold water, and applied locally. She reported that that degree of dilution helped slightly, but after experimenting with stronger solutions she ultimately used the tincture itself. 'You get an initial sting for a second and then immediate relief. You need courage but it's worth it; it's fantastic, I'd swear by it.'

She then had tried it on her young daughter in a weaker strength with gratifying results.

A convenient way to apply the tincture is to damp a pad with water, put a few drops of the tincture onto it, and as soon as the stain of the brown tincture has started to spread, press the pad on the affected part.

Many women have expressed gratitude for this advice and one reported that it helped her pruritus ani.

This is a true example of the homeopathic principle, treating like with like, even though material doses are employed.

MENOPAUSAL SYMPTOMS

Although hormone replacement therapy is a very effective treatment for menopausal symptoms, there is a significant group of women who either cannot take it, because of a medical contraindication such as previous cancer of the breast, or deep vein thrombosis, or who simply will not take it. For these women, homeopathy provides an effective alternative.

CASE 90

Mary is 57, and her menopause started two years previously. Since then she had had frequent flushes which she found embarrassing. She was hot-blooded, and always felt hungry.

I gave her *Sulphur* 30c to take as required, and she found that this effectively controlled her flushes.

CASE 91

On 22.2.80 the senior partner of a large group practice brought his 60-year-old wife for homeopathic treatment for her persistent menopausal flushes and sweats. She had had a mastectomy in 1978 for breast cancer and so hormone replacement therapy was contra-indicated.

She had five to ten drenching sweats every twenty-four hours, always worse between 8 and 10p.m., and she regularly soaked her nightclothes.

She was chilly, with a cyanotic tinge, which she said was familial, but had a dusky appearance after eating, or drinking wine. Although her hands and feet were always 'icy cold', she was intolerant to any heat, found my room too hot, took off her overcoat, and was not wearing any woollens although it was a cold February morning.

Her modalities were: worse for hot bath, worse for heat wave, worse in the morning, worse for tight clothing around neck and abdomen.

She was a tense person. Her libido was diminished 'and always has been'. Her BP was 100/80.

She did all the talking. This may not have been due to loquacity, but to her husband's attitude. He sat impassive and silent, and when, out of courtesy, I invited his comments, he replied 'I have only brought her at her request as a last resort, I don't agree with homeopathy!'

Lachesis was selected, although normally associated with intense sexual desire; *Pulsatilla* and *Sepia* were considered and eliminated.

I gave *Lachesis* 30c daily until reaction; then stop and wait.

21.3.80. She reported that the flushes were less frequent and shorter, and was pleased, but not forthcoming, and was reluctant to admit much improvement.

Then the husband spoke up: 'I kept quiet through the first interview, and have done so far today, but I have to report that I've only been asked once in the last month to put the electric fan on, and only once to leave the lounge door open. When my daughter-in-law visited recently she confided, 'Mum doesn't flap any more'. If you couldn't do any more than you've already done, I'd be pleased.'

I gave *Lachesis* 200c, to be taken as necessary.

29.4.80. She reported a severe aggravation the day after taking *Lachesis* 200c, with unprecedented bouts of sneezing. This may have been a proving of *Lachesis*. I had not met this before, but discovered Boericke mentions 'paroxysms of sneezing' (*Homoeopathic Materia Medica*, p. 388). We live and learn.

She did not repeat the *Lachesis* 200c, but reverted back to 30c, which she found she needed to take at approximately three to seven day intervals. On leaving, they presented me with a beautiful Stewart Crystal rose bowl!

Chapter 11

Homeopathy for Men

To judge by all the articles on health in the popular press, women are the only ones to suffer from diseases peculiar to their sex.

At first sight this seems a little unfair. Although there are as many men in the world as women, in the last hundred years several books on homeopathy for women have been written, together with many containing sections on obstetrics and gynaecological problems, but have you ever seen a book or chapter heading with the above title?

Sexism

Dr R.E. Ruddock was a prolific writer on homeopathy at the end of the last century. Among his most popular works were:

Ladies Manual of Homoeopathic Treatment in the Various Derangements incident to her Sex.

The Common Disease of Women, an abridgement of the Ladies' Manual.

There were other books written by eminent homeopaths about women's illnesses:

Organic Diseases of Women by Dr J.C. Burnett.

The Physical Life of Women – Advice to the Maiden, Wife, and Mother by Dr G.H. Napheys.

The Signs and Concomitant Derangements of Pregnancy by Dr W. Morgan.

The Application of the Principles and Practice of Homoeopathy to Obstetrics, and the Disorders Peculiar to Women and Young Children by Dr H.N. Gurnsey; a truly monumental work – my copy (of the 3rd edition) published in 1878 has 1,000 pages.

Thus much was written about women and children, and yet to my knowledge not one has been written specifically about men's disorders! Why?

Why?

The explanation is obvious; despite all our modern concepts about the equality of the sexes, equal opportunities and antidiscrimination laws, the sexes are different, both anatomically and physiologically; they always have been, and always will be. One unfortunate consequence is that there are many illnesses and afflictions that only women fall prey to, compared with the relatively few that only men can suffer from.

For Women

Homeopaths have consistently observed that certain medicines are indicated far more frequently in women than in men. Sometimes in the literature the phrase 'a women's remedy' appears (e.g. in the remedy pictures of *Caulophyllum* and *Crocus sativa*), or 'especially used in females'. *Gratiola* has been called 'the female *Nux vomica*'. A list of homeopathic medicines that are predominantly used in menstrual disorders includes: *Cyclamen*, *Helonias*, *Thlaspi*, *Trillium*, *Ustilago*, and *Viburnum* (which is of particular use in dysmenorrhoea). Better known, deeper-acting medicines more commonly prescribed for women are: *Lachesis*, *Lilium tigrinum*, *Murex*, and *Sepia*.

Hahnemann first discovered the use of *Sepia* by observing the symptoms of sepia poisoning in an artist friend, who was made ill by frequently licking his brush when painting with sepia pigment (which is derived from the ink of the cuttlefish). He and his colleagues then proved the remedy. Interestingly, in recording the results in his *Chronic Diseases*, among the seventy different mental symptoms listed, twice as many are prefixed with either 'she or 'her' as by 'he' or 'him'. (Hahnemann does not state how many provers were male or female.)

Men Only

There are a few diseases that are strictly limited to males, mainly affecting their genitalia, involving the prostate, testes, or penis; men also suffer from impotence. There are also some rare metabolic disorders, which are beyond the scope of this chapter, with the exception of haemophilia, to which I refer briefly on page 162.

There are also several diseases that are far commoner in men than in women, such as chronic bronchitis and lung cancer, peptic ulcers, and coronary thrombosis. Presumably, as the percentage of women smokers rises, and more women are exposed to the pressures and stresses of professional life, the predominance of men suffering from these complaints will diminish. Fewer women than men suffer from myocardial infarction, as a visit to most coronary care units will confirm. Another cause for cheer is that women's longevity greatly exceeds that of men; again, an inspection of the average residential home will emphasis this fact.

Male Preserve

We will now consider in order the illnesses that only men can acquire, and I must apologise to any male readers who may have already become a little impatient with this rather protracted preamble. I am excluding any reference to cancer since this should always be treated by conventional methods, with homeopathy only being an additional form of therapy when indicated.

PROSTATE, BENIGN ENLARGEMENT

In this distressing complaint there is certainly a place for prescribing homeopathic medicines. This well publicised disability is likely to increase as men live longer; one could even conjecture that this 'old man's disease' would overtake all men in time if they lived long enough. Happily, new non-surgical treatments are being tested, with some measure of success, including oral medication with drugs such as finasteride, but homeopaths a hundred years ago were using homeo-pathic medicines for the same purpose. Boericke lists forty medicines to treat prostatic enlargement – fourteen are in bold type. In my experience I have found the most effective one is *Sabal serrulata*, but I regard it as mandatory to eliminate any sinister pathology of the prostate before embarking on homeopathic treatment.

Sabal serrulata, when properly indicated, frequently appears to lessen the nocturnal frequency and voiding difficulties, the hesitancy, straining, terminal dribble and feeling of incomplete emptying; it also improves the flow. I prescribe it in low potency, 3c four times a day for several weeks until relief of symptoms. In early cases this is usually sufficient, though repeated short courses at intervals of three to six months may be necessary. In several instances patients have avoided having a prostatectomy by using this regime, and others have been able to postpone their operation for years.

If *Sabal* proves ineffective *Ferrum picricum* 3x should be tried, in the same dosage (see Boericke).

Kent, in his *Repertory*, has a little-known short section on the prostate gland containing a rubric 'Enlargement', with a sub-section 'senile'. I find it misleading, inasmuch as it lists *Baryta carb.*, *Digitalis* and *Selenium* in capitals, *Benzoic acid*, *Conium*, *Iodum*, and *Staphysagria* in italics, and *Sabal* only in small type. It does not even include *Ferrum pic.*, which is mentioned elsewhere in the book. In my opinion these last two should replace *Digitalis* and *Selenium*.

Where voiding difficulties are such that the man must strain, leaning forward with his legs wide apart, before the flow starts, and he feels there is a ball-like lump in his perineum, he requires *Chimaphila umbellata*. This is made from a ground holly, which rejoices in the very appropriate common name Pipissewa. I prescribed it recently to a 60-year-old man who had had all the above symptoms for the previous six months; he was quite convinced that he would need surgery. He was waiting to consult a urologist and have full investigations. After about two weeks his symptoms completely subsided and all his subsequent tests proved unremarkable. *Chimaphila* is also one of the medicines used in women with enlarged breasts due to painful tumours.

Clematis erecta is used in cases where the flow of urine is interrupted, with poor stream and terminal dribble, associated with scrotal pain, hard swollen testes and violent erections. The name of the plant will facilitate remembering this last symptom. I have also found it very useful in treating epididymitis.

Equisetum is a very useful medicine in frequency and nocturia, not necessarily associated with prostatism.

CASE 92

A 62-year-old man was complaining of frequent urging to urinate and dysuria. He was needing to get up three to four times every night (especially after drinking) for the last few years. He also had to break his journey to work to micturate, and often could not get there in time.

I gave him *Equisetum* 3c, four times a day, until reaction.

He was most impressed with the result. He had not woken up in the night once since, nor had to break his journey to work.

Again, a 73-year-old had had disturbed sleep for 'quite a while', because he had to pass urine two or three times every night. He had a good urinary flow, with no hesitancy, but frequently had terminal dribbling. He had 'no trouble in the day time'.

I prescribed *Equisetum* 3c daily until improvement. This, he claimed, had made him 'wonderfully better ... helped me a lot and stopped that lot ... and made me sleep better, for I wasn't sleeping well.'

He was able to control his nocturnal frequency for the next few years by having intermittent two-week courses of daily *Equisetum* 3c.

Other urinary problems in males also respond to homeopathic treatment, such as the following puzzling case of cystitis.

CASE 93

A 42-year-old general practitioner had suffered from frequent attacks of cystitis for the previous eighteen months. He experienced a scalding, burning terminal dysuria. The urinary flow was good, uninterrupted and virtually pain-free until the end of the act of micturition, when the pain became excruciating. Finally on occasions he would pass a white drop of ?mucus ?pus.

His full investigations, including an intravenous pyelogram and a micturating cystogram, were normal. Scans were not then available. Repeated urine cultures were consistently negative, despite the fact that he always responded to courses of ampicillin. 'It works every time. I never dare try to go through an attack without it – the pain is too severe. I have been on daily ampicillin for at least half the days of the last eighteen months, and am getting worried about possible side effects.'

He felt that his colleagues by now must regard his symptoms as of psychosomatic origin.

I discussed his case later with a leading nephrologist, who postulated that there must be an infection with an organism that had not yet been identified, but that was sensitive to a broad-spectrum antibiotic.

I prescribed *Sarsaparilla* 12c four times a day, as he was just starting another attack.

A week later he reported that he was 75% better and 'rather impressed'. I increased the potency and prescribed *Sarsaparilla* 30c, three doses at intervals of twelve hours.

Ten days later he claimed he was 80% better – he had only had the scalding pain twice in the last fourteen days and then it was mild. Previously it was severe and recurred virtually every alternate day. He had not taken any ampicillin since his first consultation.

Six months later he was 90% better, and had not taken any ampicillin or other antibiotics in that time.

Much useful information can be found in *Pointers to the Common Remedies* No. 7, by Dr M.L. Tyler, which covers cystitis, enuresis, retention and renal disorders. I have found this series of pamphlets invaluable; I used to keep a set on my surgery desk, another in my visiting case, and a third set at home, and I still use them for reference.

BRUISING AND TRAUMA OF THE TESTES

Arnica initially, followed by *Hamamelis* if the testes become increasingly painful, hot and inflamed.

ORCHITIS

When associated with parotitis (mumps), (an unusual complication which I only have seen in adults, as far as I can recall), *Pulsatilla* is most likely to be the remedy.

OTHER CONDITIONS OF THE TESTES

Torsion, hydrocele and undescended testes are surgical conditions and necessitate early surgical intervention. Although the old homeopathic textbooks give advice on how to treat them, with lists of appropriate medicines, in my opinion it would be folly to depend on homeopathy alone, and negligent on the part of any doctor to withhold obtaining a surgical opinion. The same applies to the treatment of syphilis and gonorrhoea. In the pre-antibiotic era treatments were inevitably restricted and limited in their efficacy. A hundred years ago surgery was in its infancy, and crude at best. Thus it would have been reasonable for the early homeopathic masters to give the advice they did, as conventional treatment could have been hazardous.

IMPOTENCE

There are many medicines listed for the treatment of impotence, simply because they produced impotence in the volunteers who 'proved' them, that is, who took them experimentally, in small daily doses for several weeks. Kent classifies the disorder in the section 'Genitalia, erections wanting (impotence)'. The first-line medicines in bold type are: *Caladium*, *Calcarea carbonica*, *China*, *Conium*, *Lycopodium*, *Medorrhinum*, *Nux vomica*, *Phosphorus*, *Selenium*, *Sepia* and *Sulphur*; and in most cases the choice of which medicine to prescribe would be determined by the mental, general and particular symptoms of the patient. For example, it is relatively easy to distinguish a *Calcarea* type of patient from a *Sulphur* type.

In situations where the constitutional medicine is not clear-cut (and this is often the case) it would be appropriate to use:

Agnus castus, especially if the genitals felt cold, and libido was completely lacking.

Caladium, again, if the organs feel cold, but are swollen and relaxed, if there are painful erections without desire, alternating with desire with relaxed penis, with frequent nocturnal erections and emissions leaving the glans swollen and painful. *Caladium* also is reputed to modify the craving for tobacco: I have prescribed it on many occasions for that purpose, but without significant success.

Conium, where desire is increased, but the ability to perform is diminished.

Similarly, *Selenium* is useful where libido is high, but performance impaired, as in the case of a 40-year-old male who had been impotent since being in a Japanese prisoner-of-war camp. In view of the long period of debility, with mental and physical exhaustion, I gave him *Selenium* 6c three times a day until reaction. After two weeks he reported to say that for the first time in two years he had been successful. I might add that it had been the third remedy that I had tried on him – the first two had made no difference – and thus obviating the criticism that it had been a placebo response. He remained functional, only requiring an occasional 30c dose.

Where impotence is a prominent feature in the Chronic Fatigue Syndrome, either *Phosphoric acid* or *Picric acid* will probably be needed.

There are nearly forty other medicines listed in italics for treating impotence and I have only picked out those that I have found to be the most useful.

In my experience *Lycopodium* is the medicine that has been the most often indicated and given the best results; but *Lycopodium* will only work when the patient is a *Lycopodium* type.

EXCESSIVE LIBIDO

Before leaving the subject of male sexuality I would like to make one further observation. I have read somewhere, but cannot trace the author, that the women of certain Indian tribes were in the habit of lacing their husband's drinks with small amounts of toad poison, to cool their ardour when they became too amorous and demanding! (I am not suggesting anything, but must warn you that it is most important to choose the right amphibian, because it has recently been reported that a tropical frog has been discovered that contains enough poison to kill a hundred people!) *Bufo* (homeopathic toad poison) would not work – in fact any action would be to increase libido, as *Bufo* is used to treat impotence. Alternatively, the wife might consider whether she needs a dose of *Sepia*, to help her to respond!

Kent deals with excessive libido in men in his section, 'Genitalia, male sexual passion excessive', and 'violent'. Surprisingly *Phosphorus* is one of the most important listed, along with *Cannabis indica*, *Cantharis*, *Picric acid*, *Platina*, *Silica*, *Tuberculinum*, and *Zincum*. In the case of women the condition is called 'nymphomania', and is included under 'Mentals' and not under 'Genitalia, female'.

LOSS OF CONFIDENCE AND FEAR OF FAILURE

This is another disability that particularly affects men and especially professionals, though I have very occasionally met it in women, where *Lycopodium*, when indicated, can give considerable relief. A case will illustrate this:

CASE 94
A 58-year-old dentist, renowned for his expertise in fitting bridges and crowns and to whom his colleagues referred their difficult cases, suddenly found that he had completely lost confidence in his ability to continue working. Although he had done the same sort of work very successfully for years, he had suddenly been overwhelmed with the fear that the work he was about to start would be a failure: 'There has always got to be a first time.' He agreed that in the past he could 'almost have done it blindfold', but now things were totally different. He had to check and re-check every stage of his work, he lay awake worrying about the problem, developed flatulent dyspepsia, and lost his appetite. Often he came home in the evening feeling ravenous, yet a few mouthfuls satiated him so that he could not finish the meal. Understandably he became morose, depressed and irritable, and he felt exhausted both mentally and physically. Yet when each patient's treatment was completed the patient invariably was delighted, and he was surprised with the excellent results.

He was a typical *Lycopodium*, tall, stooping and angular, with a constant frown that made him look worried. 'I was born with a frown. No, that's not true, I used to have a fantastic sense of humour, but now

I get irritated if anyone tries to make me laugh.' He confessed to being a conscientious worrier, perhaps the most specific mental symptom in the *Lycopodium* remedy picture. To add to his burden of worries he had become impotent, having premature ejaculations and failure of erections.

After taking *Lycopodium* in high potency (10M), he improved sufficiently to resume his work confidently and happily; his other symptoms settled, and his sexual performance was restored.

Had *Lycopodium* not worked when so clearly indicated, I would have offered to treat him with medical hypno-relaxation, which is a very effective alternative, though more time-consuming.

HAEMATURIA

CASE 95
Another case where *Lycopodium* worked extremely well was in a 52-year-old man with haematuria.

He first attended on 22.6.82, having suffered from haematuria continuously for the previous three years. He had been investigated intensively at a leading Birmingham hospital by the senior urologist, and all tests to discover the underlying pathology were unremarkable. Apart from passing blood in his urine every time he micturated, the patient was asymptomatic. The surgeon had prescribed continuous antibiotics for the whole of this time. Eventually, as the condition was unaltered, he was told that there was no further treatment available, and was asked, 'Can you live with it?'

The patient stated that his 'urine was always red, sometimes very red, exceptionally red.'

He had features in his make-up that indicated his constitutional medicine was *Lycopodium*, so I gave him a single dose of *Lycopodium* 200c which he took at the time, and placebo (sac lac), one tablet to be taken daily.

He returned ten weeks later (1.9.82) and insisted (his wife confirmed the observation) that after six days his urine began to clear, and was completely clear in fourteen days. 'It was quite dramatic.'

He had kept his last six-monthly hospital appointment a few weeks previously, and told the surgeon about his improvement. The surgeon suggested it might be due to the antibiotics working at last. He replied that he had not taken any antibiotics for the last year. 'I had stopped the darned things – they were poisoning me.' The doctor then added that if it were the homeopathic tablets that had achieved the improvement, he would like a case full of them.

He then discharged him from the clinic.

Note: In the early provings of *Lycopodium* some of the volunteer testers started passing urates in their urine, which settled as a red sandy deposit in the chamber pots. Obviously, in this case there was no question of the patient simply voiding urine laden with urates – the hospital would have discharged him after the first visit; indeed, the GP would have eliminated this possibility in his surgery and would never have referred the patient for further investigations.

HAEMOPHILIA

At the beginning of this chapter I make reference to haemophilia, where there is a hereditary deficiency of Factor 8, causing a bleeding disorder.

Although transmitted by females, it usually only affects males. The cornerstone of treatment is in controlled replacement of Factor 8 to prevent life-threatening bleeding, which may be spontaneous, as well as from trauma. Dr Mollie Hunton recorded six patients to whom she gave additional homeopathic medicines, following which some aspects of their health improved in each case and they appeared to have needed less Factor 8 (*British Homeopathic Journal* 1993; 92:96).

....

In summary and conclusion, these are some of the situations where homeopathy is peculiarly suitable for the forgotten sex.

Chapter 12

Musculoskeletal Disease

GOUT

When I am short of time, I am always torn between giving a conventional medicine, which I am sure will alleviate the symptoms, or making a spot diagnosis of the homeopathic remedy, and prescribing that instead. Hahnemann, you may recall, had some strong things to say in *The Chronic Diseases* about the casual, indiscriminate prescribing of homeopathic medicines on insufficient indications:

> A physician not willing to take this trouble ... and who by means of these general indications dispatches one patient after the other, deserves not the name of true homeopath. He is a mere quack, changing his remedies every moment till the poor patient loses his temper and is obliged to leave this homicidal dabbler. It is by such levity as this that true homeopathy is injured.

I accept the rebuke, but admit to being guilty of the crime on occasions. It might be better not to use a homeopathic remedy at all, rather than to use it in a hit-and-miss fashion. On the other hand, the results are so rewarding with homeopathy if the choice does happen to be correct, that one feels tempted to let the patient have the benefit of the gamble.

CASE 96
One such case was a very healthy, active and industrious man of fifty-five years who had rarely needed medical help in the twenty years that I had been his GP. I was called to him urgently on 9 September 1970 (a Wednesday), as he had been awake all night with intense pain in the first metatarsophalangeal joint of his left foot. The pain had been – and still was – hot, burning and throbbing, and he had had to uncover his foot and leave it above the bed clothes in the cold night air to obtain some relief from his pain.

He was now sitting in a chair, with his foot uncovered and elevated on a stool. The least movement or jar caused agony. The dorsum of the forefoot was diffusely pink and shiny. There was considerable local heat and he could not tolerate warmth, pressure, or any covering. There were no constitutional symptoms; as far as he was concerned, the attack had come 'out of the blue', there being no history of trauma or of gout in himself or his family.

Anyway, here was a man with a hot, shiny, painful, swollen toe joint – clinically a case of acute gout. As I had no time to take his mentals or generals, but as he had very characteristic particulars, I compromised and gave him *Belladonna* 30c alternate hours until reaction, and a prescription for phenylbutazone 200mg, every four hours, as a second string.

I called next day, and found his foot worse than the previous day. He had again been awake all night with pain; the red blush had spread further over the forefoot, and the pain now extended up to the ankle. Having a little more time, I discovered that he was a warm-blooded man normally, who in summer lay on top of the bedclothes and in winter put his feet out of bed occasionally to cool them, and who often took his shirt off in the house. I told him to continue his phenylbutazone, and took some blood for biochemical investigations. Still not being sure of the simillimum on this occasion, I refrained from prescribing a further homeopathic medicine.

I called the third day (Friday) and found him totally incapacitated and distressed with the pain. He was now unable to bear any weight, even on his heel. The burning was 'really hot' and the pain excruciating. Again he had been awake all night, despite taking full doses of phenylbutazone and liberal quantities of codeine tablets.

His blood results were now available:

Serum uric acid – 79mg per cent (Normal 1–45)
R.A. latex – negative
Blood urea – 29mg per cent

At this stage I could not leave him to suffer any more. On the very marked modalities of 'Better for cold application; worse for movement; worse for heat; worse for pressure of bed clothing; worse at night', I gave him ten pilules of *Ledum palustre* 12c, to be taken alternate hours initially, and every four hours on improvement. (This was despite the fact that he was a hot-blooded person, and that the foot was red, and not pale.)

On Monday morning (the sixth day) he drove to the surgery and walked cautiously into my room, wearing a soft shoe. He reported that he had had a very severe aggravation, coming on progressively as he continued medication. For once I had omitted warning of the possibility of this, as I had not anticipated it, so he took the whole course. 'The whole of the foot swelled up,' he said, 'and the pain got worse during the next day, so I kept on with the pills every second hour, as it was not improving.'

During this time, he sat with his foot elevated and protruding through the back door, which opened on to an entry, so that the cold wind could keep it cool. This helped to ease the gnawing, throbbing pain. On one occasion, he missed his step, jarring his heel, and the pain nearly made him faint. By Sunday, 13 September, the day after his last dose of *Ledum*, the pain, swelling and redness had virtually subsided and there was a dramatic improvement and, for the first time, he was able to wear a soft shoe and walk round the house.

He had not needed, nor taken, any conventional drugs since he first discontinued them.

On the Wednesday (the eighth day) he again attended, walking easily, and able to bear pressure over the affected joint, which was still stiff and 'aching very mildly'. I gave him one dose of *Ledum* 200c, and a few spare pilules to be taken only in the event of a relapse.

He took a second dose of this higher potency two days later (tenth day). A week later (seventeenth day) he was so much improved that he returned to work, not having taken any more *Ledum*, nor any analgesics, nor a uricosuric agent. Three weeks later (16 October 1970), another identical attack started, and this time I gave him *Ledum* 10M, every four hours until reaction. The attack, to his great surprise, subsided completely after the second dose, and he continued at work.

I do not ever remember such a severe attack of gout settling so quickly. What was even more gratifying was the fact that it had not responded to full (or even double) therapeutic doses of phenylbutazone and salicylates (one of the standard therapies in those days).

Discussion

Why didn't I give *Sulphur*?

The patient was hot-blooded – he put his feet out; the pains were burning; and he was worse at night and worse for the heat of the bed.

However, *Sulphur* pains are better for movement and better for warmth.

Clarke, in his *Dictionary of Practical Materia Media*, states about the generalities of *Sulphur*:

'The majority of the sufferings appear, or are worse, at night, or in the evening; and also during repose; when standing for a long time, and on exposure to cold air. They disappear on walking, on moving the parts affected, and also in warmth of a room; but the heat of the bed renders the nocturnal pains insupportable.'

Hahnemann states that *Ledum* is suitable, for the most part, only for chronic maladies in which there is a predominance of coldness and deficiency of vital heat.

Clarke and Nash state: 'For complaints of persons who are always cold and chilly.'

Kent states: '*Ledum*, like *Lachesis*, is mottled, puffed and bloated in appearance; there is venous stasis and constitutional coldness.' Then he adds: 'Again, we see the other extreme, where the whole body is over-heated, and the head also is in a great state of great heat.'

Ledum is like *Pulsatilla* – the two remedies that want their feet in very cold water. *Ledum* 'has a besotted look, like the face of an old drunkard. *Ledum* counteracts the effects of whisky and takes away the craving. It is to whisky what *Caladium* is to the smoking habit' (Kent). *Ledum* is listed by Dr Gibson Miller as a hot remedy in small italics.

I think the answer is that *Ledum* is a cold remedy in chronic gout; but that in the first attack, as in this case, it can still be indicated in a hot-blooded person, as events showed.

Ledum has copious, clear, low specific gravity urine during attacks of gout, and quantities of sandy deposit of various colours in between attacks (Lippe, verified by Kent).

PSEUDOGOUT

CASE 97

A 47-year-old quantity surveyor had suffered from 'pseudogout' for twenty-two years, originally confined to his left ankle, but involving his left knee for the last five years. His rheumatologist explained to him it was not true gout, because although crystals of uric acid were recovered from the joint fluid when his ankle was aspirated, there was no hyperuricaemia during his attacks of acute arthritis. A recent X-ray established that the joints were unaffected. During each attack the ankle became swollen, red, hot and tender, and the pain was so excruciating that 'in my distress I would bang the floor and cry out with pain.' It was impossible to bear weight through the joint, and pressure or movement were intolerable. The onset was sudden: his last attack a week previously began at 3 a.m., starting 'as if I had sprained my ankle', and the heat of the bed was unbearable.

For the last nine months on average he had had an attack each week, and had stopped playing golf five years previously because he could no longer walk the required distance. He still swam. An anti-inflammatory drug helped somewhat.

He was 17.2m (5ft 8in) tall, weighed 70kg (154lb), was a non-smoker, liked sunny hot weather, and felt better in the morning. Cold applications best eased his hot rheumatic pains. My prescription was:

> *Ledum* 200c one dose immediately, repeated at four to seven day intervals as required.
>
> *Ledum* 3c every fifteen minutes in acute attacks.

A month later he reported having had a severe aggravation within forty-eight hours of taking his first dose of *Ledum* 200c. The ankle pain became significantly worse, and the exacerbation lasted nearly a week. At the same time a similar pain started in his right ankle, but this settled within hours. Taking *Ledum* 3c every half hour slightly modified the pain. He continued taking *Ledum* 200c, at seven-day intervals, each time provoking a shorter and less severe aggravation, followed by a gradual remission. The last aggravation only lasted four hours. He already felt very much better in himself. He had only taken two anti-inflammatory tablets in the previous three weeks, which was unprecedented for months.

I suggested that he reduce the frequency of *Ledum* 200c to seven to fourteen day intervals and try *Belladonna* 30c every quarter hour if another flare-up occurred.

Three months later he was '80% better, back to golf, regularly on the driving range, and on one occasion have managed a complete round.' When asked if *Belladonna* helped in an attack, he replied, 'I haven't had occasion to try it – I've not had any heat in the joints since I saw you last. I ran 150 metres to catch a bus in heavy rain recently; it's a long time since I last ran anywhere. Before that I had to hop along.' He had not taken any anti-inflammatory drug in the last four months, nor had a single flare-up of his joints. 'I'm still improving.' He was quite sure his improvement was entirely due to the medicine.

Although his pain modalities – worse for pressure and movement – pointed to *Actea spicata*, the strong temperature modalities – burning pain better for cold – in an arthropathy that started in the feet and then extended up to the knees, indicated *Ledum* to be the simillimum.

OLECRANON BURSITIS

CASE 98

One Saturday morning in July 1993 a local doctor who had had no previous experience with homeopathy phoned me for advice about his 'olecranon bursitis'. He said the hot burning pain in his elbow joint had kept him awake most of the previous night, and that he had had to sit up in bed with his arm in a sling, applying cold packs to his elbow to get any relief. An X-ray had failed to show any significant change in the joint, and his serum uric acid was not raised. He had been taking maximum doses of paracetamol without much benefit and he stated he was intolerant of all the main non-steroidal anti-inflammatory drugs.

On questioning him it transpired that the bursa was not grossly swollen; certainly not enough to warrant aspiration, or to cause him severe pain. He considered the lesion must be periarticular, and he did not feel that antibiotics were indicated.

He had heard of *Rhus tox.*; could that help?

I outlined the indications for using *Rhus tox.* and some of his modalities fitted: i.e. stiffness after immobilisation, with the first movements predictably the most painful. However, he found relief from cold applications – not hot – and was not unduly restless.

I considered *Ledum*, which is often indicated in acute attacks of gout, but the arthropathy usually commences in the feet and spreads upwards.

Belladonna seemed an obvious choice, as the bursa was hot, both objectively and subjectively.

I then asked him to describe the pain: was there any stinging sensation, like that of a bee sting? He replied that that exactly described it, so I suggested he obtained *Apis* 30c from our local chemist, and take it every hour initially, reducing the frequency as improvement occurred. If this proved ineffective he should then try *Belladonna* 30c at fifteen-minute intervals as required.

He phoned me two days later to thank me for the great relief that followed using *Apis*; the joint was settling satisfactorily, and he had not needed *Belladonna*.

POLYARTHROPATHY

CASE 99

A 43-year-old female school teacher had suffered from a non specific polyarthropathy for four and a half years. She was seronegative. She only obtained relief from her pain by taking an anti-inflammatory drug twice a day. *Pulsatilla* seemed to be indicated:

- Her symptoms were changeable – the pain flitted from joint to joint.
- The joints swelled and became hot, but not red.
- The pain was made worse by rest, better by cool, better by movement in bed and unaffected by pressure.
- She could not 'tolerate the sun'.
- She had flushes and sweats, and had to change her night dress at least once a night.
- She was thirstless.

Accordingly I gave *Pulsatilla* 30c x 1, followed by *Pulsatilla* 6c three times a day until relief.

A month later she referred to 'the wonder pill' she had taken. She was able to play golf the next day, the first time for months. She had had better nights, and had cut her dose of the anti-inflammatory by half.

Treatment

    Pulsatilla 10M x 1
    Pulsatilla 6c as required.

Five months later she relapsed, after having been able to discontinue the anti-inflammatory completely for three weeks. *Pulsatilla* no longer helped her. However her symptoms had changed significantly:

Her legs were restless at night and jerked; she could only control them by lying on her stomach. Her hands and feet burned and itched intolerably. 'I could scratch them off.' The soles of her feet were sore and the heels and metacarpophalangeal joints were tender. She had tried *Rhus tox.* without benefit. I considered *Zincum met.*, which often controls restless legs, but decided *Medorrhinum* was more appropriate, as it covered all the above symptoms.

Admittedly she did not have the modalities – made better by damp weather (she now was unaffected by weather), made worse from day-light to sunset, and she had not had occasion to determine whether she was better at the seaside. It proved to be the simillimum at the time, illustrating how it is necessary to change the medicine when the symptoms change during the course of an illness.

ARTHRALGIA

CASE 100

19.1.72. Mrs W. consulted me, complaining of 'rheumatic pains' in the right shoulder and the interphalangeal joints of the first and second fingers of her right hand: worse before damp, worse at rest; better in the warm and unaffected by movement. She was not sure about the pains being bad on the first movement after rest, and then she added, 'Isn't it strange all my pains are on the right side?'

She was small, ginger-haired, very cold-blooded; better in the warmth generally and locally.

Treatment

Rhus toxicodendron 200c x 1

26.1.72. No improvement. On closer questioning she said it was worse twenty-four hours before rain, no better when the rain came. Worse before snow. Worse in the cold.

Treatment

Rhododendron 12c three times a day, until reaction.

3.2.72. Took two doses, at 10a.m. and 2p.m. Omitted 6p.m. dose because her pains were definitely worse. By next day the pains had eased considerably and she remained pain-free for two complete days. Then relapsed and took one dose; and found she needed one approximately every second day.

On questioning, she was not worse before a storm nor before thundery weather, which is usually very marked in a *Rhododendron* case. However *Rhododendron* seemed to be suiting her and she also displayed some forgetfulness, which is present in the mentals of this remedy. She continued with a 12c dose when necessary.

OSTEOARTHRITIS

CASE 101

Bertha was a 73-year-old widow with severe arthritis of the left hip and knee following a fracture of the left femur. Her complexion was rather dirty white with a sallow tinge, and she had warts on her face. She was rather depressed. She had been housebound for the last five years and required continuous phenylbutazone (or equivalent).

21.8.71. Pain worse in hot, dry weather; better in the damp weather. Better for the warmth of bed.

Treatment

Causticum 200c when necessary, at not less than two-week intervals. Given six doses.

16.10.71. Very great improvement. Still one pill left.

CASE 102

A 54-year-old female secretary developed painful osteoarthritis in the interphalangeal joint of her right hallux following trauma some years previously. The condition had deteriorated during the previous two years, and a fortnight before she saw me an orthopaedic surgeon had put her on his waiting list to have an arthrodesis, as the only way of alleviating her pain. The joint was swollen, red and tender and she had to wear a flat shoe one size too large on the affected foot. She had had to stop ballroom dancing, which she loved, and had become irritable and impatient with clients.

She described the pain as 'a gnawing toothache, twenty-four hours a day.' The pain was:

- Unaffected by time, cold or warmth, or pressure.
- Worse for wet, movement, walking.
- Better for rest.

She was 15% overweight and still added sugar to her drinks. Her treatment included:

Reducing her sugar intake.

Bryonia 200c every fourteen days as required.

Bryonia 3c four times a day on the intervening days until improvement.

Two months later she claimed that the *Bryonia* definitely helped to ease her pain, and that when she stopped taking it her toe burned and throbbed more.

I switched medicines to a trial with *Actea spicata* 6c four times a day until improvement.

Six weeks later she said, '*Actea* is definitely the better of the two medicines. It takes a day to work, but is more effective than any of the drugs my doctor has given me. Initially, if I stop taking it the pain returned within a day. Now I can go for several days between short courses.'

I asked her if she had had any side effects from the medicine. 'Yes, if I take it for too long I get a sickly pain in my stomach, as if I had been kicked.'

By reducing the dose of *Actea* 6c to three times a day, and by shortening the courses of treatment she found she could control both her arthritic pain and the abdominal side effects of the medication. When I last heard from her she said she had deferred the proposed surgery indefinitely, and added, 'I can now wear shoes with heels.'

This patient apparently 'proved' *Actea*; she developed stomach symptoms which she had never had before, but which had been experienced by volunteers who first tested this medicine to establish its subtoxic properties. Boericke describes the stomach symptoms as: 'Tearing, darting pains in epigastric region with vomiting, etc. Cramp-like pains in stomach and epigastrium, etc.'

In contrast, an aggravation is a stirring up of symptoms already present. It is most unusual to get an aggravation, let alone a proving, from low potencies.

Among the most useful homeopathic medicines for treating arthritis the following four exemplify distinguishing pain modalities.

	Movement	*Pressure*	*Touch*
Actea spicata	worse	worse	worse
Bryonia	worse	better	worse
Radium bromatum	better	better	
Rhus tox.	better	better rubbing	worse

One would expect a tender, painful joint to be sensitive to, or worse from, touch, but for it to be eased by pressure or movement is unexpected.

Comment

Actea spicata is prepared from the root of the baneberry plant, and like *Actea racemosa* (also known as *Cimicifuga*) is a rheumatic remedy. It is specifically indicated for arthritis of wrists and ankles and the small joints of hands and feet. The two significant modalities are that the joints swell and become tender after slight use or exertion, and that the severe pain is worse for cold, cold weather, movement and touch, and better for rest.

EXOSTOSES

CASE 103

In December 1994 a retired 70-year-old headmaster developed severe pain in his left shoulder when moving his arm, particularly when elevating it beyond the horizontal position. As he was left-handed this disability became a real handicap.

The pain progressively increased, necessitating taking full doses of painkillers and non-steroidal anti-inflammatory drugs (NSAIDs): despite this medication he was wakened repeatedly at night by any movement that resulted in putting pressure on the shoulder.

An X-ray of the shoulder showed 'a reasonably normal glenohumeral joint, some subacromial bone changes, with some soft tissue calcification'. The radiologist suggested a diagnosis of 'impingement syndrome and possibly rotator cuff damage'.

After two months suffering he saw an orthopaedic surgeon, who diagnosed supraspinatus tendinitis and injected the shoulder with a long-acting steroid. This afforded considerable relief, but only for two weeks, so a month later he had a second steroid injection, which again only alleviated his pain for a fortnight. The surgeon then ordered a scan, but unfortunately the patient had to wait nearly five months for this. The scan revealed an unrecognised exostosis. Accordingly the surgeon put the patient on the urgent waiting list for surgery. Precisely at that time I prescribed *Calcarea fluorica* 30c at seven-day intervals, and 3c four times a day on the intervening six days.

After one month on *Calc. fluor.* the pain had lessened sufficiently to warrant deferring the operation for another month. The operation would have involved considerable protracted post-operative pain, and total immobility of the left arm for at least a month, which to a left-handed person would be an added trial: it also would preclude him driving his car. I then prescribed a trial of *Hecla lava* 12c twice a day for four days in place of *Calc. fluor.*

The result was most encouraging, so that he continued taking *Hecla* for the next month until his operation date arrived. Again, with the surgeon's consent he deferred the operation, and three months later was taken off the list.

Nine months later he had regained full free active use of his left shoulder and was not taking any analgesic or NSAID, and his shoulder no longer disturbed his sleep at night. He had discontinued taking *Hecla* altogether about a month previously.

While all this was going on he developed a very painful tender left hallux, which was attributed to an ingrowing toenail. A podiatrist performed a wedge resection, but the pain and tenderness at the terminal phalanx continued, actually increasing so that he had to sleep with a cage over his foot, as the least touch even of a sheet was intolerable. X-ray of the toe revealed an exostosis on the side of the bone, and further surgery was advised.

It was just at this time that the patient switched from *Calc. fluor.* to *Hecla* for his shoulder pains.

When the operation date arrived his toe was so much improved that he could squeeze it without pain, and even knock it; he could even wear ordinary shoes once again. As it no longer hurt him or bothered him the podiatrist agreed to leave the toe alone, and it remained asymptomatic until his death from a vascular accident three years later.

Hecla is made from the finer ash from Mount Hecla falling in distant localities, and the ash from this volcano contains silica, alumina, lime and magnesia, with some oxide of iron. According to Clarke, sheep in the vicinity of Hecla had immense exostoses on the jaws. The finer ash which fell on pastures at a distance was the most deleterious; the gross ash near the mountain was inert. In cows, post-mortem examination showed the intestines filled with ash, hardened to a mass; and several young horses died from lumps on the jawbones, so large as to cause dislocation. In sheep the bones of the skull, jawbones, and thigh and shin bones swelled and bulged. Clarke further states that 'Clinical experience has shown the power of *Hecla* to arrest many forms of bone disease, including osteosarcoma, tubercular and syphilitic osteitis and exostoses.' He then adds most significantly 'The swellings amenable to it are painful and sensitive to touch; worse from touch and pressure.'

RHEUMATISM

CASE 104

8.6.68. Kathleen, aged 62 years, was complaining of 'rheumatism' in her shoulders, knees and thumbs. She was unable to hold shears or clip hedges for more than a few minutes because of this.

Her pains were unaffected by movement or wet weather, but were possibly worse in dry weather.

She was not painful or stiff first thing in the morning. She could not tolerate heat or cold. She craved cheese.

She felt that her knees were very cold. She had aching varicose veins and piles.

Treatment

Cistus canadensis (Rock rose) 30c, 2 doses at 12-hour intervals. To be repeated in one week if required.

26.8.68. Telephoned: 'Miraculous'. In two days she was better and able to mow two lawns and cut a long hedge.

Cistus has in its materia medica, 'sensation of coldness in various parts', 'worse slightest exposure to cold air', 'desire for cheese'.

RHEUMATOID ARTHRITIS (RA)

Rheumatoid arthritis is a most unpleasant, debilitating and often progressive disease. Conventional drugs are used that are extremely powerful, often with very unpleasant and even dangerous side effects. Often the relentless advance of the disease is not even stopped by these powerful drugs. Some cases are described below that have been modified, or improved remarkably, by the judicial use of homeopathic remedies. That is not to say that homeopathy can help all cases of rheumatoid arthritis. Even the most experienced homeopathic physician will be defeated by this disease on occasion.

CASE 105
Mrs A.B., age 47.

Her rheumatoid arthritis began eight years earlier, when she was thirty-nine years old. It progressed so rapidly that within a year she started on prednisolone which she has taken ever since. Despite this her condition continued to deteriorate, and her husband installed a lift in the house when she could no longer climb the stairs. She became dependent on a wheelchair and her husband adapted a van, which allowed her to travel without getting out of her chair.

At her first consultation she was maintained on prednisolone 5mg and indomethacin 50mg daily.

Her homeopathic prescribing features were:

Both her joints and she as a person were intolerant of hot weather. Her joints became hot and throbbing in hot weather, and stiffened after prolonged immobility, such as occurred during the one-and-a-half-hour road journey involved in coming to see me. First movements were painful, but her limbering up time was only fifteen minutes, presumably shortened by her steroid therapy.

She had tried *Rhus tox.* in potency without benefit; hardly surprising because *Rhus tox.* has a marked aggravation from cold, not heat.

Her general modalities indicated *Pulsatilla*, rather than *Sulphur*, so I prescribed *Pulsatilla* 30c at seven to fourteen day intervals as required. Two months later she reported a considerable improvement:

'My joints no longer become hot and throbbing.'
'I can manage without the home help now.'
'I can peel an apple and cook my own bread; I can even slice bread – the first time for years and years.'
'I can now sew.'

She found the first dose of *Pulsatilla* 30c lasted two weeks and the second dose nearly three weeks. She continued for the next few years taking intermittent doses at three to four week intervals in addition to prednisolone.

A year later she began to get 'jumpy legs', which wakened her and made her sit up and sit on the side of the bed. The problem seemed to occur most often when she wanted to micturate, and she found her legs flexed and moved more than she could voluntarily make them move. The attacks came by day as well, and she said: 'On one occasion I nearly jumped out of my chair, because I was leaning forward at the time. I can't get out of the chair unaided normally.'

She started taking *Lathyrus* 3c four times a day and found it controlled the legs satisfactorily. At my suggestion she switched to *Cuprum* 30c (which is often very effective for controlling cramps), but her 'jumps' returned. 'I stuck it for three days, but had to revert to *Lathyrus*, and that stopped them.'

She had not dared reduce the dose three months later, because whilst taking *Lathyrus* she slept so much better. I persuaded her to reduce the dose to one a night if she felt at risk, and for the following year she took *Lathyrus* 3c when necessary, as well as her conventional medication. The last time I saw her she said, 'My legs don't plague me now at night.'

She could no longer stand, and her prednisolone had been increased to 8 mg daily, yet both she and her husband were adamant that the homeopathic medicines still worked, and had vastly improved her quality of life.

CASE 106

A 46-year-old motor mechanic developed rheumatoid arthritis in March 1976, which rapidly involved 'every joint' of his body. He was seropositive and his rheumatologist had tried various different anti-inflammatory drugs but was unable to control the pain. He therefore took additional soluble aspirin, on occasions taking fifteen in a day, but had to reduce this high dose as it caused tinnitus and affected his hearing. A short course of steroids had been very beneficial, but had not been repeated.

He was understandably very concerned about his future, because his mother had developed rheumatoid arthritis at the same age, and had spent the last fifteen years of her life totally dependent, in a wheelchair, not even being able to feed herself.

A further concern was that his job was a heavy one; singlehandedly he maintained a fleet of twelve lorries. This was very hard work and involved straining his shoulders, elbows, wrists and fingers all day long, and these were his worst affected joints. He foresaw that soon he would have to change a job he enjoyed and was trained and qualified to perform.

He had had to stop rock-climbing in the Alps, and dancing – which had been his favourite pastime for twenty-three years, and for which he had won many awards.

He was determined to keep going, and felt somehow he could work it off, rather than rest it off. He tackled jobs that inevitably made his joints swell and stiffen, knowing it would take three to five days for them to recover. He argued that it 'rebalanced them'. He had reached the stage where 'I couldn't walk across a carpeted floor. I took three minutes to get out of my car at work and limber up to walk past the office window. I was so embarrassed, walking like a man in plaster.'

25.7.76. He had been off work for the past week, but his joints were no better for the rest.

His symptoms were:

Joints made better by the cold, and cold applications, and better for movement.

Generals (in himself): made worse by heat, hot baths, summer, evenings, the heat of the bed; he exposed his feet to cool them down.

He admitted he was an aggressive, competitive person who could speak his mind, and 'blow his top'; not 'the placid sort'. He had a hearty appetite, and could eat all foods, including fat.

Treatment

Sulphur 200c split dose, i.e. three doses in one day.
Continue conventional medicines.
Seriously consider changing to lighter work.

26.8.76. For the first three days after *Sulphur* 200c he had an aggravation (which I had forewarned him might happen). Within a week he was walking with his dog for two and a half hours on the Clent hills (his previous limit had been ten minutes). 'I flew at things, starting to dig the foundations for a new patio and wheeling full barrows of heavy wet earth. After two days of digging I got a reaction and had to slow down. I still can't believe it, and I'm dead scared it will all have to relapse.'

He attended out-patients in the meantime, where it was decided he could defer starting the gold injections they had anticipated he would need, as he had improved so much. He still needed the anti-inflammatory, but had reduced his aspirin intake considerably.

Treatment

Tuberculinum 1M x3 (split dose). (His aunt had died of TB when she was in her early twenties.)

22.9.76. Still improving. Has managed to dance for five minutes without a setback.

Treatment

Sulphur 10M x 1

11.11.76. Pronounced aggravation the same night he took *Sulphur*, followed by a skin rash which lasted two weeks. He never had had a rash like this one, or any rash since childhood. He felt low for the first three days, and then 'fantastic'. He increased his workload, working from 8.30 a.m. to 7.30 p.m., not getting home until 8.30 p.m. He found he could grind valves for several hours, go for forest walks 'over ankle-rolling ground', and resume dancing. He had been discharged from hospital because of his improvement. His RA latex titre was then 64, which was significantly raised.

Treatment

Sulphur 10M (x3 in split dose).
Reduce the anti-inflammatory and aspirin.

10.2.77. Just completed two weeks of very heavy work, servicing the two largest vehicles in the fleet. Dancing for half an hour once a week.

28.2.77. Relapsed and off work for the past week because joints so stiff.

Treatment

Sulphur 10M x3 (split dose).

5.4.77. Very much better after three days.

Treatment

Sulphur CM x3 (split dose) (experimentally).

6.6.77. Involved in serious car accident on holiday, when his car was written off and he was 'badly jarred and shaken up'. A very severe relapse followed: all his usual joints flared up, and new joints were involved. *Sulphur* eased slightly. *Pulsatilla* 3c alleviated significantly for a few months, but it was only when he reverted to steroids in December that he got symptomatic relief.

His arthritis became so severe that he was unable to work for three months and lost his job. He started gold therapy, which had to be discontinued because of renal toxicity.

He could no longer dance, because his ankles were 'collapsing'. Neither *Radium bromatum* nor *Causticum* helped (given because of the modalities of his arthritic pain), and he became increasingly disabled.

I last saw him three years after his first consultation. He was anaemic and had developed haematuria. This was attributed to a nephropathy caused by the anti-inflammatory drugs rather than the gold injections. He was ambulant and could drive his car, but was unemployed. He was maintained on prednisolone.

In all, a disappointing sequel to a promising start. So what went wrong?

Obviously the car accident stirred things up, but I still feel that his joints must have suffered unnecessary damage from the excessive strains imposed on them during his work. Maybe the developing nephropathy was disturbing his immune system, vitiating the action of the homeopathic medicines. I wish I had been more forceful in insisting that he changed to a more sedentary job earlier in his illness. It may not have made any difference, but who knows?

CASE 107
A 65-year-old company director developed seropositive rheumatoid arthritis which particularly affected the small joints of his wrists, hands, feet and ankles, and to a lesser extent his knees and shoulders. The arthritis progressed rapidly, and within a few years he was taking 10mg prednisolone daily, and two tablets of a non-steroidal anti-inflammatory drug.

He was still attending the Birmingham Queen Elizabeth Hospital each month as he was under the surveillance of a rheumatologist, who for seven years had included him in a hospital-based research study on RA. He had tried all the usual first-line drugs, and also on several occasions had tried reducing the daily dose of prednisolone, without success. He had had several intra-articular steroid injections, which only afforded temporary relief.

The patient's disability depressed him, particularly because he could no longer play more than a few holes of golf at a time – and golf had been his life for many years. He said that, after gripping his clubs for a short while, 'I could have cried with the pain in my wrists.' Also the distance he could walk was strictly limited because of the pain that developed in his knees. Some of his symptoms were typical of *Rhus tox.*, inasmuch as the pain was:

Worse for cold.

Worse in the mornings.

First movements were most painful, better after limbering up.

This suggested that *Rhus tox.* might be the indicated medicine, but the pains also were better for pressure and better for rest.

Treatment

Medorrhinum 30c single split dose (i.e. three doses taken in one day).

Bryonia 3c four times a day to follow.

Medorrhinum is used for chronic rheumatic conditions, especially when the legs feel heavy and the patient cannot keep them still, and the soles of the feet are tender and sore. The ankles and knees are often involved. I have discovered that using a concurrent low potency for local pathology does not apparently interfere with the action of the appropriate main remedy.

Six weeks later he reported that he was no better. I then gave him *Actea spicata* 3c four times a day until reaction, i.e. either better, or worse, with instructions to discontinue at this point and resume it when needed. I told him that if he had an initial aggravation which was only attributable to the medicine, it was likely that improvement would follow. Six weeks later he attended for review.

'There has been a vast improvement. I can see my knuckles again for the first time in a long while, and I can't remember feeling so well and so free from pain for years, even in the days when I was on 25 mg prednisolone daily.'

He could grip his golf clubs firmly without precipitating intense pain, and he was not afraid to shake hands with anyone.

'I played golf last week and managed fourteen holes. It was drizzling and the ground was heavy. I fell on my backside in the mud for a start. Normally on hard ground the most I ever manage is nine holes, and that is not often.'

He continued his prednisolone 10 mg daily and *Actea* 3c four times a day.

A month later he was regularly playing sixteen holes in a day. However, three weeks previously he developed severe epigastric pains accompanied by belching. He stopped taking *Actea* and these symptoms disappeared.

Over the following months he continued to improve, taking intermittent short courses of *Actea*, and succeeded in gradually reducing his daily prednisolone to 7 mg.

CASE 108

(This case was not diagnosed as rheumatoid arthritis, but as 'synovitis' as she remained rheumatoid factor negative. However I think she should have been correctly diagnosed as 'seronegative rheumatoid arthritis'.)

Mrs M.J. was a bank clerk who first consulted me on 5.6.91, complaining of arthritis of her feet of eighteen months' duration, and recently of pain in her left wrist and fingers. She was forty-one years old, 1.63 m (5 ft 4 in) tall, 57 kg (126 lb) in weight, and had never smoked.

She described the pain in her feet 'as if the arches had dropped'; the pain was 'crippling', and had only been temporarily helped by physiotherapy. She derived some comfort from wearing special insoles in her shoes. An orthopaedic surgeon had injected cortisone into her metatarsophalangeal joints, but the relief from pain had only lasted for three weeks. She had seen a rheumatologist privately who had eventually eliminated a diagnosis of rheumatoid arthritis, and diagnosed 'synovitis', as her blood was seronegative on three occasions; and her latest blood test in February 1991 revealed that her ESR (erythrocyte sedimentation rate) had dropped from 31 mm/hr to 25 mm/hr. She also had developed iritis, but this subsided after six weeks treatment with eye drops, and had not returned. She partially controlled the pain with anti-inflammatory drugs, four times a day, which she had taken for the last year.

In the past she had been very athletic and active, playing squash weekly, running, and regularly enjoying ten-mile walks. For the last year she had 'been crippled' and had had to discontinue all these activities. Her left hand ached if she attempted icing a cake or arranging flowers.

Her past history and family history were unremarkable. She had no known allergies, nor had she suffered any untoward reaction from vaccinations. She had never suffered from dermatitis.

She suffered from PMT, worse on the second day of menses.

Modalities

The pain was of a burning aching character, especially after walking.

'My feet go red hot with the pain, as if on fire. I often put them in cold water.'

Worse on rest.

Worse on waking in the morning.

Better for movement.

Better for applied warmth, yet occasionally her feet were better when moved to a cold part of the bed.

No change in the damp.

First movements after rest were painful; the joints were stiff, better for limbering up.

She herself was chilly, loved heatwaves, bruised easily, was worse for cold winds.

No change in thunderous weather.

No other relevant homeopathic prescribing features were elicited.

At this stage I shortlisted, and then eliminated: *Medorrhinum*, *Ledum*, *Apis*, and *Actea spicata* as the required medicine, though each had some good indications for choosing it, as the following abbreviated summary of their indications for use reveals:

Medorrhinum: Lameness and stiffness of larger joints. Severe rheumatic pains in extremities, tenderness and soreness of soles of feet, rheumatism of wrists with loss of power. Restless legs.

Pain worse for warmth, damp, draughts, thunderstorms, sunrise to sunset.

Better uncovering feet in bed at night.

Ledum: Rheumatism begins in feet and travels upwards. Always chilly yet warmth of bed intolerable. Small joints of feet hot, swollen and pale. Soles painful – can hardly walk on them. Worse at night, for the heat of bed and for motion. Better for cold, and putting feet in cold water.

Apis: Joints of hands and feet swollen and red. Burning, stinging pain. Worse for touch, pressure, heat in any form.

Better for the cold, uncovering and cold bathing.

Actea spicata: Rheumatism of wrists, fingers, ankles, toes. Joints swollen and red.

Worse for touch, least movement, pressure, and after exertion.

The obvious choice was *Rhus tox.*, except that she was not worse in damp weather.

This need not necessarily contraindicate *Rhus tox.*, although it is included in Margaret Tyler's list of rheumatic medicines about which she states: 'Unaffected by change of weather excludes: *Dulc.*, *Nux m.*, *Phos.*, *Ran. b.*, *Rhod.*, *Rhus tox.*, *Sil.*, *Tub.*'

However, it is not in her list 'not affected by wet excludes: *Calc.*, *Merc.*, *Nat. s.*, *Ruta.*'

I therefore prescribed:

Rhus tox. 30c twice daily at intervals of 4–14 days according to response.

Nux vom. 30c for her PMT (worse cold wind, worse second day).

A month later, on 8.7.91, she returned to report that she had had an aggravation of her pain the day after taking her first dose of *Rhus* 30c. It lasted two days, and on the second day she had had to visit London. This involved a considerable amount of walking, which predictably had increased her pain. Her second dose, four days after the first, did not produce an aggravation but, she said, 'after it there was a tremendous difference; the pain was greatly reduced. I felt a lot better, and was able to walk freely, with no swelling of my feet. I inadvertently forgot to take my anti-inflammatory tablets, and had no relapse. I have only taken two a day instead of four since then. I'm so amazed; I can curl my toes up, whereas previously there were many days when I couldn't move them at all.'

She then told me about a serious side effect.

After the first day's doses of *Rhus* her skin began to itch all over:

'It was a dreadful itch all over my body, arms legs, trunk, neck, everywhere. It started the morning after the first day's treatment and lasted day and night for a whole month. It looked like a heat rash; it wasn't blisters, only blotches, where I had scratched. I could only ease it slightly by applying cold flannels constantly to my skin.'

In answer to my questions she told me that the itching was temporarily aggravated after the second dose of *Rhus tox.* 30c taken after four days (taken because the improvement of her joint pains had come to a standstill).

She had not taken a subsequent dose in the last three weeks.

She had never experienced anything like this before, or had any skin problems in her life.

On close questioning she could not identify any likely cause other than the *Rhus tox.*; there were no emotional or stress factors involved, nor food intolerances or known allergies. She was insistent that nothing different had occurred in her routine apart from the homeopathic medication.

After about a month the irritation was at last beginning to subside.

Because her joints were so dramatically improved she elected to have a higher potency of *Rhus tox.*, rather than an antidote, such as *Anacardium* (which produces skin eruptions very similar to those caused by poison ivy).

I gave her *Rhus tox.* 1M, single dose.

On 5.8.91, a month later, she was able to report that the itching skin had not flared up after the taking *Rhus* 1M, and that it had finally settled completely ten days later.

She was delighted with her progress.

'I am 75% improved, and can claw my toes up for the first time for a year. I still don't think the damp weather makes any difference.'

Treatment

Rhus tox. 6c twice daily as required.

A month later (9.9.91): She had returned from a walking holiday, having regularly done ten-mile walks. She had played two games of squash in the last fortnight, and resumed running, and 'things I could never have done before I came in June.'

She only had mild burning or aching at the end of the day, at about 8 p.m., unless she had walked more than five miles earlier in the day.

She no longer was compelled to immerse her feet in cold water to ease the burning. She did not like walking barefooted in the morning, not because the floor was cold, but because her joints were still slightly stiff and painful to move on waking. She immediately put on her slippers with special insoles, and was able to mobilise her joints within a few minutes.

Asked how much she felt she had improved in the last two months, she replied, '70%, and I am still improving. If I didn't improve any more I could accept this, and wouldn't bother to go to a doctor about it.' She still didn't find that damp weather affected her, or her joints.

6.11.91. 'Feeling fine. Not taken *Rhus tox.* in the last six weeks.'

Comment

Rhus tox. would appear to have been the simillimum, because of her marked improvement, after an initial short aggravation. Her violent skin reaction must be attributed to a proving of the remedy, and is most unusual following a single dose of *Rhus tox.* 30c.

We tend to think of *Rhus tox.* as a rheumatic remedy, although its skin and bowel symptoms are equally prominent and important.

Rhus poisoning causes the most intense unbearable itching of the skin, probably as much as any other plant, and can produce severe erythema, vesication, urticaria and erysipelas, which have persisted for six weeks after exposure to the plant in sensitive subjects. It is worth reading the account, given by Hughes in *A Manual of Pharmacodynamics* (pp. 779–80), of a lecture on the toxicology of *Rhus tox.* at the Medical School of the Westminster Hospital over a hundred and fifteen years ago. Hughes observes, 'I have thought well to write this account from an author not partial to the homeopathic doctrine, as I shall have to show that the efficacy of *Rhus* as a medicine is displayed in the very regions in which it is so active as a poison. We shall see it as a remedy for many cutaneous affections, for rheumatism, and for typhoid conditions of several kinds.'

CASE 109

On 23.2.72 a 67-year-old man attended evening surgery, apologising that he had been unable to come to a morning surgery, which in those days finished at 10 a.m. Although he only lived a hundred yards away, he had tried unsuccessfully for the last three mornings, but his stiff painful joints had not loosened up in time.

As a young man he had lived in Malvern and had cycled daily the twenty-five miles each way to the Rover factory (then the Austin Motor Company), where he worked.

He had all the typical appearances of early rheumatoid arthritis, involving the knuckles and wrists of both hands, and particularly the proximal interphalangeal joints of his fingers. He also complained of severe pain in his right shoulder and both knees, which had deprived him of sleep for the last two nights. After settling comfortably in one position he found that just as he was dropping off to sleep his knees began to ache so intensely that he had to shift his position and turn over. When he finally managed to settle off to sleep the pain woke him within an hour, forcing him to change his position again. In the early hours of the morning he would finally drop off into a more prolonged sleep, but on waking found the pain more excruciating, and his knees, wrists and fingers locked on trying to move them for the first time.

These first movements were the most painful, and it took him nearly two hours to get dressed. He found relief by immersing his hands in very hot water as he tried to mobilise his fingers. Once he had limbered up and freed his joints, he could keep the pain and stiffness at bay throughout the day if he constantly kept them moving. By evening he was so exhausted that he was glad to sit and watch the television, but the immediate benefit was short-lived, as the gnawing pains returned and increased the longer he kept still.

I made a mental note that the weather had been unusually wet for the last week, whereas the patient had found that cold weather was far more upsetting than wet weather; later he developed a definite aggravation in wet weather. He certainly was better in warm surroundings, and his joint pains were reduced by applied heat.

He had attended my partner two weeks previously, again at an evening surgery, and been prescribed analgesics and indomethacin, but his condition had deteriorated rather than improved.

I prescribed stronger analgesics and gave him a single pill of *Rhus tox.* 1M. I also asked him to try and come to a morning surgery if possible, in a couple of days, but he said there was no hope of that, because he couldn't get there in time. 'It takes me ten minutes to come down the stairs, and I have to put a screwdriver through the ring of the key to open the back door.' However, he agreed to try. Two days later he attended the end of morning surgery asking, 'What is in that miracle pill?' He had had 'marvellous sleep' for the last two nights, and the stiffness and pain on waking in the morning had steadily improved, so that he was able to get dressed without much difficulty that morning. He had not needed any analgesic tablets, and already the swelling and stiffness of his joints was noticeably diminishing. It was raining at the time he came, yet despite the damp he felt much better.

I prescribed placebo (sac lac) tablets.

22.3.72. He attended morning surgery again. He had had a slight relapse in the last few days, having been gardening and decorating in the previous weeks, neither of which he could have contemplated attempting a month previously.

Treatment

Rhus tox. 1M x 1 and sac lac, one every morning.

I explained that the pill I gave him (*Rhus tox.*) contained the powerful active medicine, and the daily placebo tablets that he got on prescription were back-up tablets, to enhance the action of the stronger pill.

He returned two months later, having maintained his improvement until the last few days, when his symptoms relapsed, and asked for another 'bomber', as he correctly surmised that the effect of the last pill was wearing off.

Treatment

Rhus tox. 200c x 1. Placebo daily.

Two weeks later he was back again, and this time I gave him:

Rhus tox. 1M x 1.

From then on, for the next four years he attended approximately every two months – to be precise he had twenty-three doses in thirty-eight months. He only came when his condition deteriorated.

On 1.7.72 he stated:

'Within a fortnight of the first dose in February, I had lost the cramp in my toes. I could walk for miles, when on occasions previously I couldn't get out of my chair unaided. I mended a puncture on my grandson's bicycle without tyre levers. I was up a ladder decorating the outside of the house [I had seen him doing this] and sleeping quite well. The different pain tablets I tried when my pains began to return did not really help, so I came for another "bomber".'

I experimented with different potencies of *Rhus tox.*, trying 30c, 200c, M, 10M, CM, and on one occasion MM. Contrary to my expectation and current teaching, there did not appear to be any extra duration of action when using the highest potencies – all potencies above 30c seemed to give equal benefit.

In general, low potencies (3x to 6c) are short-acting and have to be repeated frequently, and the more accurately the patient's symptoms match the remedy picture (i.e. those symptoms produced by the medicine, when taken in repeated subtoxic doses by healthy volunteers), the higher one prescribes the potency.

The patient had two aggravations, one following a 1M potency, and the other after a 10M – this was unusual, as he had been using *Rhus* in these potencies for two and a half years. The first aggravation followed taking a pill that was manufactured in 1949, and thus was twenty-five years old – suggesting that potencies keep their strength for years.

I was able to confirm that camphor can apparently antidote a homeopathic potency, as taught by the early homeopaths. On 13.1.76 I gave the patient a pill of *Rhus tox.* 1M, and at the same time a pill of sac lac medicated with tincture of camphor. He returned three weeks later, on 4.2.76, to report that he had not improved at all since his last dose. I told him it was a pity he had waited so long before returning, but after a repeat single dose of *Rhus* his joints quickly settled again.

I presented him at a course on homeopathy for doctors at a Birmingham Hospital on 1.5.76. A rheumatologist who was present was somewhat sceptical about the patient's diagnosis, and asked to see his recent X-rays and blood tests. He agreed with the radiologist's report:

'Hands and wrists: There is periarticular rarefaction of the bone and some narrowing of the joint space. No erosions are detected. The appearances favour early rheumatoid arthritis.'

Rose Waller Titre:

February 1974	256
July 1974	512
April 1976	128

A level above 32 was considered diagnostic of rheumatoid arthritis in those days.

I understand that the patient survived six more years, managing adequately on infrequent doses of *Rhus*, without recourse to strong conventional analgesics or non-steroidal anti-inflammatory drugs. He then died from an intercurrent infection.

Chapter 13

Skin Problems

Arsenicum album

Some of the well-known homeopathic medicines are called 'poly-
chrests', because each one can be used to treat a number of different
conditions. Prominent among these is *Arsenicum album*, white arsenic,
best known to the general public in fact and fiction as a deadly poison
obtained from weedkiller. It has had other uses; apparently the arsenic-
eaters of the Tyrol used to condition themselves, by gradually increasing doses, to tolerate up to six grains (360 mg) every two days (fatalities
have followed the ingestion of 100–300 mg in people not so
conditioned).

These Styrian mountain dwellers maintained that it imparted a sense
of invigoration and enabled them to carry enormous loads up steep
mountain passes. They assumed that since they were vegetarians they
needed arsenic to strengthen their muscles, to help them digest their
coarse bread and potatoes and to improve their breathing.

When Hahnemann decided to investigate the homeopathic use of
arsenic he needed to know the side effects and toxic effects of the
substance. There was no shortage of published articles to which he
could refer; indeed, in his literature review he discovered eighty
authors who had written on the subject. He then experimented on
himself, his wife, and six other doctors, testing (proving) the effects of
taking repeated small doses of arsenic, each one keeping an accurate
log diary of their symptoms.

These volunteers thus established a remedy picture of arsenic, based
on the predictable side effects that the majority of any healthy group of
people would develop if they continued taking small doses of arsenic
for long enough.

Hahnemann had to battle against the practice of his times of
administering large doses of highly toxic drugs like arsenic, quinine
and mercury to patients who subsequently died from their treatment
rather than from their disease. Yet this 'heroic' medicine was acclaimed
by the doctors of those times, who stoutly defended their methods.

As recently as 1941, *Martindale's Extra Pharmacopoeia*, which included a full description of the toxic effects of arsenic, stated that:

1) Arsenic could be given as a general tonic; it was one of the few substances deserving of the name, because it increased the weight and strength of the patient in wasting diseases such as tuberculosis, and neurasthenia with malnutrition.
2) In treating disseminated sclerosis (multiple sclerosis), most neurologists considered arsenic as the most useful drug.
3) Arsenic held an important place in the treatment of chronic eczema.

Nowadays I could agree with some of those statements, but only if they were referring to the use of *Arsenicum album* in potency. Any therapeutic benefit derived from using material doses of arsenic as prescribed in Martindale's would be because – unwittingly – the medicine was acting homeopathically, i.e. 'treating like with like'. The homeopathic principle depends on the law of similars – not opposites, as in conventional medicine – and small doses are not essential, although in practice they are more effective and produce less side effects.

Let me amplify this in the case of eczema. Repeated small doses of arsenic can produce an exfoliative dermatitis which nowadays could be diagnosed as eczema. In my 1961 'formulary' of the Birmingham Skin Hospital the section 'Mixtures' includes Liquor Arsenicalis (Fowler's Solution) with a maximum dose of up to 5mg white arsenic per day! Nowadays this would be regarded as a toxic dose of arsenic, which is known to accumulate in the body and can be detected in the hair and nails months, and even years, after it has been taken. Yet this medicine was frequently prescribed to be taken in the treatment of chronic eczema.

Arsenic can produce, and therefore cure, other skin lesions apart from eczema; such as urticaria, psoriaform scaly rashes, and herpes with vesicles that burn intensely, especially at night. An interesting letter in the *British Medical Journal* (27.1.79) records that:

In 1900 an extraordinary number of cases of 'alcoholic paralysis' were admitted to the Workhouse Hospital in Manchester, and many of these had herpes zoster (shingles). Septimus Reynolds, a physician of the Manchester Royal Infirmary, remembered that 'arsenic was the only drug that produced herpes'. He immediately tested the local beer for arsenic content, and found it to be present. The arsenic was eventually traced to the sulphuric acid used to convert cane sugar to invert sugar required for brewing, and with its removal the epidemic ceased.

In chronic cases *Arsenicum album* is invaluable, especially in skin conditions, eczema alternating with asthma, neuralgias, renal failure, left ventricular failure (cardiac asthma), when homeopathic medicines can be taken in addition to conventional medication.

It best suits people who are neat, tidy and fastidious; in Kent's *Repertory* only *Arsenicum album* and *Nux vomica* are listed under 'fastidious'. I remember a patient telling me that if she thought she was dying, and the mantleshelf in the bedroom was dusty, she would have to get up and dust it – 'I couldn't die peacefully until it was dusted!'

ATOPIC ECZEMA

CASE 110

A man of forty-five had suffered all his life from atopic eczema of the hands, and had attended Birmingham Skin Hospital for over thirty years. A six-week course of medical hypnorelaxation helped him to control his itching, and in his own estimation did more good than the thirty years hospital treatment, but he still needed Betnovate (betamethasone) cream and polythene gloves for occlusion for the next three years.

He then suffered from a recurrence of his intolerable burning, itching rash on the palms of both hands. I decided then to use homeopathy, and found that he was always chilly, always liked heat and the fire, and always had a reputation for 'keeping up a fug'. He was very fastidious. At work, his hands irritated so badly that he used to go to the washroom and put them in very hot water – 'a lovely feeling' – or if available used an electric fire to ease the irritation.

He was given *Arsenicum album* 30c, followed a week later by *Arsenicum album* 200c. First the vesiculation and later the irritation ceased, and he remained more or less symptom-free for the next three years, with only an occasional dose of *Arsenicum album*. He discontinued all topical therapy.

This case illustrates the use of Dr Gibson Miller's list (page 15), as both the patient and the remedy, *Arsenicum album*, were extremely 'cold', and the rash had the marked modality that, although burning in nature, it was eased by the application of intense heat. This is a rare and peculiar feature of white arsenic.

CASE 111

A 31-year-old lady was seen at the Birmingham General Hospital by a consultant dermatologist in 1965. He noted that she had eczema of the atopic type, which had troubled her on and off since childhood, and was associated with hayfever and occasional asthma. He treated her with the conventional treatment of the time, namely calamine cream and a potent steroid ointment for her face.

The skin did settle over the next few months, but flared up badly following a minor accident in February 1970, when she injured her ankle.

She required full doses of antihistamines, but was still kept awake by the irritation, and found her condition unbearable. By May she required short courses of steroids, which she said 'Calmed it down a bit and stopped it oozing, but left the skin red and flakey.'

In mid-May she developed cystitis with gross bilateral oedema of the legs, which required diuretics. She remained normotensive, but complained of blurred vision. By now, the affected parts of her skin were cracking and oozing, and her face was becoming involved. The rash was located in the flexures (elbows and knees), and in the axillae, and she looked a pitiful sight. She was also becoming acutely depressed about her condition, and saw no hope for the future. The exudate was watery and transparent, and the cracks were deepening.

She felt cold and could not keep warm. In appearance, she looked a typical *Pulsatilla* type, and as *Graphites* is a complementary remedy to *Pulsatilla*, I gave her *Graphites* 30c, twice daily until reaction. (29.5.70).

She reported 'almost immediate relief' of the itching, and took doses twice a day for the next two days, during which time the skin gradually improved. On the third morning she 'forgot all about her pills' but had to take one that evening as the rash was much worse.

I saw her a week after her first dose, when an unbelievable transformation had taken place, and she was delighted. She had had no more *Graphites* since that fifth dose, four days previously, but was given some more to take if necessary.

Since atopic eczema is an intractable condition, for which steroids are often required, this recovery seemed to me remarkable, especially as steroids had failed to relieve.

I reviewed her on 15.8.70, when she had some residual eczema limited to the wrists and between the toes. She had been taking one dose of *Graphites* 12c whenever her lips or outer skin of the canthi of the eye lids started to crack, which was approximately every third day.

It is notable that there was no aggravation here, a problem that is common in the treatment of eczema. It is vitally important that the administration of the remedy is stopped as soon as there is a reaction –

whether positive or negative – and in this way aggravations should be avoided.

This patient illustrated well the constitutional type of *Graphites* – corpulent, chilly, costive, cheerless, catching colds. They have unhealthy skin which festers, and oozes a honey-like, sticky exudate. It complements *Pulsatilla*.

SCALP ECZEMA

CASE 112
A male university student was complaining of severe crusting of his scalp, which caused severe itching, involuntary scratching all night and bleeding. I gave *Oleander* 30c, one dose, which gave complete relief for one week. A second dose cleared the condition entirely.

Oleander is particularly indicated for eruptions at the margins of the hair, with violent itching, bleeding and oozing. The skin is very sensitive, with the slightest friction causing soreness and chapping.

SUN SENSITIVITY

CASE 113
A 3-year-old boy who suffered from eczema was also very sensitive to the sun; even short exposures made his skin 'burn' and his eczema flare up. For the previous two years his mother had had to protect him each summer from strong sunshine, keeping him indoors or in the shade, both at home and when on holiday. In those days (1975) effective sun barrier creams had not been formulated.

I gave him *Antimonium crudum* 3x tablets (which are grey!) three times a day for one week (see Boericke).

His mother reported that they seemed effective, so I increased the potency to 12c alternate days.

She returned two weeks later to state that they were so effective that he had been able to play outside each day in the hot sunshine without any adverse reaction. She and her husband were mystified, but delighted. I observed that during the previous fortnight there had been a heatwave, and Birmingham had had the hottest day for fifty years, and for seven consecutive days the temperature had been over 27°C (80°F). She responded: 'And he was out in all that.' They both ascribed this achievement to the homeopathic medicine. 'It must have been those tablets, he could never have done it otherwise.' She then added that they had spent a day at Burnham-on-Sea, and recalled that last year when they went there her husband had had heatstroke ('He can't stand the sun'). He had tried all the available creams with no success. This year 'He tried some of our son's tablets, and they worked with him. It was so hot I had to stay in the shade.'

Antimonium crudum 200c weekly protected both father and son for the rest of the hot weather.

CASE 114

Similarly, a middle-aged man had suffered from severe sun dermatitis for six years. He could not expose his skin to the sun for more than fifteen minutes without it burning intensely and forming pustules. His previous doctor had tried virtually every known treatment, including antihistamines, barrier creams, courses of injections, and cortisone.

When he consulted me, I suggested that he saw a leading Birmingham dermatologist, and, as an interim measure, gave him *Antimonium crudum* 12c to go on with. Within a week he could face the strongest sunlight and had bathed in trunks all day during a short heatwave. He had even been in the greenhouse and to the seaside in an attempt to produce a rash to show the specialist, but without any success!

The dermatologist wrote to me, 'Since your last pills, the above-named patient has been completely immune from sun dermatitis. I should be extremely interested to know what these pills are.'

I had a long and interesting discussion with the specialist, who could not understand how antimony sulphide could work, as it was not mentioned in any dermatological textbook!

I explained the difference, and told him that the best way to test the effectiveness was to wait and see how long the cure lasted.

As I had anticipated, the patient returned to report that his sun dermatitis was coming back again. His first dose had relieved him completely for nine weeks. I gave him one dose only of *Antimonium crudum* 30c, which I anticipated would ease him for some months to come.

CASE 115

Finally, I had another middle-aged man who was very keen on his allotment and a keen grower. Gardening was a problem, as he had developed a severe sun sensitivity ever since coming back from the Far East, where he had been during the war.

For the previous five years he had also been unable to grow

tomatoes, or even handle the plants, on account of irritation and blisters that developed on his skin.

Rhus tox. did not ease his sun dermatitis, but *Antimonium crudum* did. I gave him the 12c potency three times daily for four days, and he was most impressed with the way the blisters cleared. It was then that he mentioned his tomato sensitivity to me, so I gave him *Solanum lycopersicum* (tomato) 30c, one pill twice a day for six doses, and he went through all that summer without any reaction, despite growing tomatoes again.

I repeated the treatment the following year, although I am not sure that he really needed it.

ACUTE URTICARIA

CASE 116

The husband of a 41-year-old woman rang me to say that she had had severe diarrhoea and vomiting all night, after eating some tinned food the day before. It was now settling on *Arsenicum alb.* from the Home Remedies kit, but she was covered from head to foot with 'nettle rash', causing frantic itching.

I ordered *Urtica* tincture, 10 drops in a glass full of cold water, to be used as a compress.

When I visited at 12 noon she was asleep. Her mother, who had collected and applied the *Urtica*, was amazed. The patient said, 'The relief was instantaneous. It was amazing, it took all the sting and burning away immediately. I have never felt such dramatic relief.' The weals also subsided very quickly so that now there were just very small urticarial spots remaining over the whole body.

ACNE ROSACEA

CASE 117

Rosacea is an unpleasant condition which is treated conventionally, not very successfully, with long-term antibiotics.

My patient was a 31-year-old woman who had developed rosacea nine months earlier, following her first confinement.

The rash was burning, and was aggravated premstrually and by sunshine, external heat, wind and on waking each morning. She could not tolerate tight clothing around her neck or waist, nor a hot bath or shower. Despite this marked aggravation from heat, she was a chilly person.

I gave four doses of *Lachesis* 30c, one to be taken each morning until improvement.

Two weeks later she returned; the relief had been dramatic. She had used her last dose, and the burning was returning. It had been quiescent all the day time since starting *Lachesis*, and was only minimal on waking.

She felt better, and said people had commented on her improvement. Surprisingly, she could now bear tight clothing, and a hot bath.

I prescribed *Lachesis* 200c, to be followed by *Lachesis* 10M if and when her condition relapsed. Over the next few months her face cleared, but she required intermittent doses of *Lachesis* for the next few years.

ACNE VULGARIS

This is an equally distressing condition which affects teenagers, causing much embarrassment and lack of self-esteem. Again it is treated conventionally by long-term antibiotics, causing a problem with antibiotic resistance.

Kali bromatum is in bold type in Kent under 'Face, eruptions, acne', but I have had little success with it.

I discovered *Natrum bromatum* listed under treatment of acne in *Homoeopathic Therapeutics* by Lilienthal, but I cannot find it in any of the repertories. I use this very successfully in cases of acne associated with the *Natrum* type of personality and a greasy skin.

Other useful medicines are *Calcarea silicata*, *Hepar sulph.* and *Silica* – all in bold type in Kent.

SUPPURATIVE CONDITIONS

CASE 118

A 30-year-old man who had recently joined my list attended a morning surgery, and declined to sit down as he was in too much pain from his pilonidal sinus, which had flared up a week previously. It was his twenty-first relapse in thirteen years, and despite the extreme pain and tenderness he was emphatic that he was not going to have further surgery.

'I couldn't stand another operation. Even after surgery it takes weeks to heal.'

That was why he had put off coming to see me, in case I insisted on referring him to hospital again.

The lesion was red, angry and inflamed, like a boil that needed lancing, and was exquisitely tender. It had remained unchanged for the last week.

I gave him *Hepar sulph.* 30c to be taken cautiously, every four hours until the sinus discharged effectively. He returned two days later. The 'boil' had come to a head and discharged the same evening, with no further increase in pain, and was subsiding satisfactorily. This was unique in his experience, and he observed that I had not even prescribed an antibiotic. I told him to stop taking *Hepar sulph.* and gave him a single dose of *Silica* 200c.

The condition cleared up, so that he did not have a further relapse to my knowledge during the next five years that he remained in the village and on my list.

In my experience, *Hepar sulph.* should be used cautiously as it can accelerate the inflammatory process too rapidly, causing unnecessary distress. It should be used when suppuration appears inevitable, in order to 'ripen' the boil or abscess, and should be discontinued as soon as it is discharging freely.

Silica has a well-earned reputation for healing after the discharge has subsided. It suits chilly, sweaty people, with cold extremities, who overclothe because they are intolerant of cold and draughts, and have unhealthy skin; such was my patient.

VARICOSE ECZEMA

CASE 119

Grandma H. was an old, broken-down, bowed woman who hobbled round the village in her bedroom slippers, as her callosities were too painful to allow her to wear ordinary shoes. She had had varicose eczema for years, but no oedema and no cardiac failure.

I saw her first on 26.11.71 – for two months she had a varicose ulcer on her right shin, for which she initially used Cetavlex (cetrimide cream). For the last fortnight the district nurse had been calling and cleansing the affected area with Aserbine cleanser and applying Aserbine cream (malic acid).

The day before I saw her, she had been woken at 4 a.m. with burning and stinging of the ulcer, which necessitated her taking her bandages off and liberally applying more cream. The whole shin was purple in appearance, almost necrotic-like dry, glistening skin. The ulcer area was approximately 2 cm (¾ inch) in diameter. The surrounding area was not tender to touch and painless by day.

The patient could not tolerate external heat, so I gave her a dose of *Lachesis* 12c (at twelve noon) and a second dose to be taken the next morning.

The following day the district nurse reported that the patient was delighted. She had had her first uninterrupted night's sleep for weeks.

Two days later, there was a slight relapse of stinging. I gave *Lachesis* 200c x 1.

CASE 120

A 74-year-old obese, diabetic widow had become virtually housebound on account of her bronchitis, angina and arthritis. Her dyspnoea limited her walking to less than fifty yards without a rest; she was often too breathless to talk, and on occasions she spent the night sitting in her armchair, on account of her orthopnoea. She was hypertensive and hypothyroid. Her diabetic retinopathy prevented her from reading the markings on her diabetic syringe accurately.

She was currently under the surveillance of an eye surgeon, a chest physician and a consultant who specialised in treating diabetes.

Her daily cocktail of medicines included co-proxamol, thyroxine, an ACE inhibitor, frusemide, isosorbide dinitrate and an antacid. She also used bronchodilators, both salbutamol and a corticosteroid in metered aerosol inhalers, a corticosteroid metered dose nasal spray, and frequently had courses of antibiotics for her chest.

She had developed a large and painful refractory varicose leg ulcer, and since conventional applications had not helped, the district nurse tried an iodine-based one. The result was disastrous. She was allergic to iodine and the pain that followed was so excruciating that she was reduced to tears. Even after the bandage had been removed the pain continued for weeks, and despite full doses of dihydrocodeine the 'sharp sticking pains' prevented rest and sleep.

As she was an old National Health Service patient of mine, now on my son's list, I visited her and left her with a supply of *Nitric acid* 200c to be taken at four hour intervals initially, then at a reduced frequency according to the response. She found one tablet eased the pain for four hours the first day and by the third day each dose lasted about eighteen hours. Two weeks later she requested a prescription for more *Nitric acid* 200c, reporting that she had stopped taking dihydrocodeine after the first dose. She added, 'Those tablets give wonderful relief.'

What is most interesting is that the homeopathic medicine appeared to have worked despite the considerable amount of conventional medicines she continued taking. This is a lesson – not to be put off prescribing homeopathically in such a case, as the homeopathic medicine will still work in a complementary way.

ALOPECIA

Homeopathy can also work for difficult hair problems, as the following case shows:

CASE 121
Whilst working as a clinical assistant in a Birmingham hospital I regularly met another GP whose sessions coincided with mine. One afternoon he bemoaned the fact that his young wife had become acutely depressed because her hair had been coming out in combfuls for some weeks. Every night she stood in front of the mirror in tears as she observed the increased thinning of her hair.

He had taken his wife to consult Birmingham's leading dermatologist (who himself was as bald as a coot), who prescribed a six-week course of oral cortisone. This was many years ago, when cortisone had recently been newly introduced to the pharmacopoeia. The doctor was horrified at the suggestion, because already the side effects of steroids were coming to light. He asked me what I would do, if in his situation. He knew nothing about homeopathy, but realised I used it.

On questioning, it transpired that his wife had become irritable, depressed, hypersensitive to noise, and loveless. 'Her libido is at an all time low.'

I gave him a single dose of *Sepia* 200c to give to his wife. I forgot all about the matter until a week later, when I was surprised to find him waiting for me on the main steps of the hospital.

'Jack, what in the world was in that tablet you gave for my wife?'

I explained it to him, and asked how she was. 'It is unbelievable, it is like a second honeymoon; I can't keep up with her!'

On inquiring about her hair, he replied that it had stopped falling, and also her depression had lifted, and she was no longer irritable. She had not taken any cortisone.

HYPERHIDROSIS

CASE 122
A 41-year-old man who was short-built and grey-haired had been suffering from hyperhidrosis for two years.

He had had active chest tuberculosis in 1958, which was treated with conventional antitubercular drugs for three years. He had been finally discharged from the Birmingham Chest Clinic in 1970.

17.10.69. Seen on account of his excessive night sweats, at the Birmingham Chest Clinic. No significant cause discovered.

September 1970. Referred to consultant physician as 'sweats profusely each night during sleep, and sweats by day if dozes off in a chair'.

All investigations, chest X-ray, blood tests etc. were normal.

Anxiety was diagnosed and he was put on a tranquilliser – diazepam 5mg three times a day.

In October 1970 I had tried *Mercurius solubilis* 30c, one dose every three days for four doses. Nine days later I tried *Psorinum* 30c x 1 with no improvement. I regarded his symptoms as purely psychosomatic, and did not attempt any more than in a half-hearted way to explore the possibility of any further homeopathic treatment.

5.2.72. Still sweating as badly as ever. Wakes up in the early hours with his pyjamas soaked right through. Has to change them at least once every night. His head sweats to soak his hair.

I gave him *Tuberculinum* 30c x 1.

10.3.72. Reported that two days after his last medicine the sweats were controlled for nearly three weeks. He just had occasional slight sweats. He still could not tolerate heat and extreme cold. Condition as bad in the winter as in the summer. Requesting further supply. Given six doses to be used monthly, only if required.

This case illustrates that even with the apparently most intractable problems, homeopathy can afford some relief if the correct remedy is chosen.

Chapter 14

Some Interesting Cases – Anecdotal but Significant

POST-VIRAL FATIGUE

CASE 123

Mrs L.P. was a 46-year-old housewife, very conscientious, independent and hardworking. Her duties were always on top of her, keeping her up until midnight most nights. She was a tall, lightly-built, *Sepia* type, 'cold-blooded' who many times previously had benefited mentally and physically from a single dose of *Sepia* 200c.

She suffered from a chronic vaginal prolapse, and wore a vaginal pessary.

On 20.2.66, during an influenza epidemic, she developed a transient rise in temperature 37.2°C (99°F) and such profound lassitude that she had to stay in bed for several days. The flu didn't follow the typical local pattern, but dragged on; there was no history of shivering or going very hot, no marked sweating, no severe headache; but she complained of diffuse muscle pains all over the body. She commented that she had felt this coming on for over a month.

She took *Gelsemium* 30c for two doses, and then tried getting up, but after a few hours she was forced to retire to bed again, on account of weakness and the extreme heaviness of her limbs.

A week later I gave her one dose of *Picric acid* 30c, with no noticeable change. Each day she tried getting up to deal with her domestic and family responsibilities, and a few hours later had to struggle back to bed, exhausted.

On 2 March I gave her *Sepia* 200c with no effect, but in retrospect the mentals did not match this time.

I performed some investigations, as follows:

Hb: 15.0 gm. ESR 9 mm/hour. Film normal, with slight anisocytosis.
Packed cell volume: 40%.
RA Latex: Negative.
White blood count: 9,600.
C-Reactive Protein: negative.

Two days later, on the morning of 4 March, she had a severe shock on entering the room of an aged aunt (whom she had been looking after all the past winter) and thinking mistakenly that she was dead.

On 7 March she was worse, and at this juncture I felt I must do something more to help her, so I elicited the following 'mentals' and 'particulars':

Depressed; aversion to meeting visitors; irritable, even with close friends, because weak and helpless. Worse from anticipating outstanding duties that must be done. Eyes not focusing; humming noise in ears; anorexia; empty sensation in stomach. Dark yellow urine on waking; breathless on minimal exertion; profuse prostration; limbs heavy and joints aching. Afebrile since first day of illness; waking unrefreshed from sleep, with definite morning aggravation.

The mention of passing very yellow urine put me on the track of *Kali phosphoricum*, and I gave her one dose of the 30c potency.

Although I had given *Sepia*, as it was her constitutional remedy, I was not surprised it failed to improve, as she was not manifesting her previous mental symptoms of indifference to her family and profound sadness to the point of tears. Indeed, to add to her worries, she desperately wanted to be downstairs to cater for her family, and grieved the more that she was too weak to do so.

The *Picric acid* was previously given because of her 'brain fag', inability to think clearly, and heavy, weak legs.

After her single dose of *Kali phos.* 30c she didn't pass any more yellow urine. She began to improve rapidly and was downstairs much of the next day, beginning to tackle her domestic chores with returning strength and enthusiasm. Within a week she was back to normal, which is unusual in my experience in cases of reactive depression.

Kali phos. is a great remedy for neurasthenia with prostration aggravated both by mental and physical exertion. In Kent's *Repertory* it figures under the headings 'Weakness' and 'Weariness', both in heavy black type, and 'Lassitude' in italics. It is listed under 'Ailments from anger' in italics, and 'Grief', and under 'Blurred vision', 'Aversion to company'; 'Noises in the ears: buzzing', and 'Humming'.

Surprisingly, it is not included under 'yellow urine' at all in Kent, only under 'cloudy urine' and 'saffron-coloured urine' (in small type); but Boericke lists it under 'Yellow urine, dark' in italics, and it was using this repertory at the bedside that gave me the clue. Clarke describes the urine as 'saffron-coloured'.

Fortunately, in order to treat a patient homeopathically, it is not necessary to make a definitive diagnosis. *Kali phos.* would have worked in this case whether the diagnosis was post-viral fatigue or depression, because the prescription fitted the simillimum.

STREPTOCOCCIN

CASE 124

A 41-year-old radiographer was referred for homeopathic treatment. Her doctor's letter summarised her illness:

> Her main complaints are fatigue and muscle aches. Her problems started when she developed an illness consisting of fever, malaise, arthralgia, myalgia, and an urticarial-type rash. She then developed sweating and stiffness of her hands, neck pain and a sore throat. She had numerous investigations which were all rather inconclusive apart from a raised anti-streptolysin (ASO) titre. It was felt she had had a streptoccal infection with incomplete rheumatic fever. Since then she has been on continuous low dose penicillin. However she has not returned to her normal health. Her medical history prior to this event was unremarkable. Perhaps homeopathy can give her some relief.

The patient's symptoms were similar to those of post-viral fatigue. She accepted that her illness might he protracted, but her major concern was that she had already been on penicillin V 1gm daily for eighteen months, and her rheumatologist had told her emphatically the previous week that as long as her ASO titre was significantly raised she must continue taking penicillin, even for years if necessary. This disturbed her. Her latest ASO was 960.

She was a typical *Pulsatilla* patient, so I prescribed:

Pulsatilla 30c, once weekly.
Penicillinum 30c, once weekly.
Streptococcin 30c, once weekly, all on different days.

I advised her to continue taking penicillin as prescribed by her consultant. A month later she reported 25–30% improvement.

At her second monthly follow-up she recounted her latest consultation with her rheumatologist three weeks previously. He told her that her ASO had fallen dramatically to 160. 'He said he could hardly believe it, and could not explain it. I told him I was coming to you for homeopathic treatment. He replied that he couldn't really approve, but it was my decision. He then added that some of his colleagues believed in homeopathy.'

Happily he continued to give her the same considerate sympathetic attention, and six months later told her he was very pleased with her progress.

By now she was well enough to visit New York and New Orleans, to take up tennis after a lapse of twenty years, and go swimming.

Two months later her ASO titre was still down and she was living an active life again.

She continued to improve steadily over the next year, until I lost contact with her.

BRUCELLOSIS

CASE 125

A wiry, energetic 50-year-old headmaster had suffered from recurrent attacks of pyrexia of unknown origin (PUO) for the last fourteen years, starting ten years after he had returned from India. He had been very thoroughly investigated at a hospital for tropical diseases seven years previously and all the tests were unremarkable. As the attacks continued I referred him to another teaching hospital, and again a whole battery of tests were repeated, with no significant abnormalities being discovered. The hospital letter said that he was a fit-looking man, who had no rashes or lymphadenopathy; his liver and spleen were not palpable. It was emphasised that tests showed he did not suffer from brucellosis. I was advised to submit a blood sample for culture at the onset of the next attack.

The recurrent attacks of fever lasted seven to ten days and recurred three to five times a year. In the attacks he became nauseous, his body went cold, especially his knees and legs, and he ached all over the body, like flu. Following the rigor his temperature rocketed to 40.5°C (105°F), to be followed by drenching sweats, the whole cycle lasting three or four hours. About four hours later the cycle returned, so that he got through twelve pairs of pyjamas in twenty-four hours, and his bed had to be changed three or four times a night.

19.4.73. Pyrexial with rigors for 10 days. ESR 35 mm/hr. Blood culture negative.

14.6.73. Pyrexial again. Very frightened with pains in chest. Drenching sweats. Can predict within 10 minutes the time of the next rigor (every four hours).

Treatment

Aconite 30c, then *Belladonna* 30c, then *Nux Vomica* 30c.

4.10.73. Pyrexia as before. Tests all negative.

22.10.73. Typical relapse. Bright red flushed appearance.

Belladonna 30c quarter-hourly.

27.10.73. Drenching sweats without rigor or fever. *Belladonna* reduces temperature and eases thumping headaches.

Eupatorium perfoliatum 1c half-hourly (for deep bone pains).

8.11.73. *Brucella* 30c three times a day for three days, then weekly for three weeks, then monthly.

10.5.74. Never felt so well for years. No attack since staring *Brucella* 30c.

Now taking monthly doses.

10.6.74. Following his monthly dose, he woke shivering and had a very mild attack.

This was possibly an aggravation from *Brucella*. Discontinue until another attack.

12.12.75. No pyrexia for two years. He maintained this improvement for at least the next five years, until he moved from the district and I lost track of him.

Although there was no question of him having a *Brucella* infection, (repeated tests were negative), *Brucella* 30c was prescribed on the homeopathicity of his symptoms.

I learned that years later he had another PUO associated with the symptoms of acute cholecystitis and that at a subsequent cholecystectomy pathogens were isolated from his gall bladder. With hindsight, these were blamed as the probable cause of his previous febrile attacks.

This is another example of homeopathic treatment successfully alleviating symptoms when no definitive diagnosis has been established.

CONGENITAL ADRENAL HYPERPLASIA

Congenital adrenal hyperplasia (CAH) is a metabolic disorder in which, as a result of an inborn error of metabolism, there is defective synthesis of corticosteroid hormones by the adrenal cortex. CAH is inherited by the autosomal recessive mode and the abnormal gene is thought to be in chromosome six.

CAH is rare and the synonyms include: adrenogenital syndrome, adrenal virilism and ambiguous genitalia. The CAH group of the Research Trust for Metabolic Diseases in Children has only about 150 members, and the patient described here is thought to be one of the oldest persons known to have CAH.

In 95% of cases of CAH the cause is a deficiency of 21-hydroxylase (see figure below), so that the production line for cortisol stops at 17-hydroxy-progesterone (17-OH) and that for aldosterone at progesterone. The production of androgens is increased, because the deficiency of cortisol stimulates the pituitary to increase the release of adrenocorticotrophic hormone (ACTH). The clinical consequences are:

1) Androgen excess: masculinisation, ambiguous genitalia at birth.
2) Aldosterone deficiency: causes salt-losing crises in about one third of CAH patients (Collier et al., *Oxford Handbook of Clinical Specialties*).
3) Sexual precocity: accelerated growth until early puberty with premature fusion of epiphyses and short adult height.

Treatment comprises lifelong replacement of cortisol with cortisone, prednisolone or dexamethasone (DM). The dose needs to be increased at any stressful event, at which time salt losers also need urgent IV saline (*Congenital Adrenal Hyperplasia*, National Organization for Rare Diseases). Treatment is usually regulated by measuring serum 17-OH.

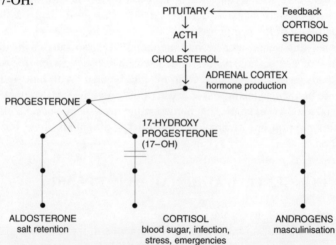

Sites of action of 21-hydroxylase in the production of hormones by the adrenal cortex

206

CASE 126

Presenting Symptoms

27.1.93. Female, aged 32, complaining of:

1) Infertility.
2) Asthma for seven years. increasing progressively. For nine months she had required a nebuliser twice daily, and routine use of salbutamol and beclomethasone inhalers.
3) Allergy to horses, dogs, cats and parrots, though not to poultry.
4) Cramps.
5) Arthropathy: most joints hurt at times. She required calipers for her weak ankles.
6) Buccal ulcers and reflux oesophagitis: was taking omeprazole (Losec).
7) Stools always loose despite taking an antidiarrhoeal agent. At times she had diarrhoea with colic which, if unchecked, precipitated a crisis.

Past Medical History

CAH was diagnosed at birth, with minor plastic surgery to her external genitalia needed in infancy. During childhood, her growth and 17-OH blood levels were monitored regularly.

Some years after marriage, she and her husband moved to a remote hill farm in south-west Wales to breed shire horses and compete at local and national horse shows.

In the nine years since their marriage, her husband had taken her sixteen times to a hospital in adrenal crisis for emergency intravenous saline and intramuscular steroids. Usually they were away from home and new to the hospital they attended. The medical staff were often reluctant to accept his diagnosis and deferred treatment until after some investigations. Despite her critical state, there was often a delay of several hours before treatment.

The crises were predictably triggered by any infection, diarrhoea (she permanently suffered from loose stools), by any emotional upset, shock, fright or accident, and by dental surgery. Her husband always carried hydrocortisone 100mg for emergency IM injection but often this was insufficient to avert a crisis.

In 1990 she became pregnant, surprisingly because she had had amenorrhoea for many years. She was booked into a London hospital and admission was recommended until the baby was viable. As she lived nearly two hundred miles away this was impractical; so she attended twice weekly, until at 24 weeks she developed asthma and pre-eclamptic toxaemia, followed by intrauterine death of the foetus.

Since she still had anovulatory infertility, it was decided to increase the daily dose of dexamethasone from 0.75 mg to 1.0 mg in an attempt to reduce her 17-OH from 17 nmol/l to 11 nmol/l. (Ovulation can he suppressed by 17-OH being either too high or too low.) She was reluctant to increase her steroids, as her weight had steadily risen from 69.9 kg (154 lb) to 89 kg (202 lb) and she was only 1.5 m (4 ft 11 in) tall. At this stage, she decided to seek a homeopathic opinion.

History of Presenting Symptoms

Despite taking a maintenance dose of DM 0.75–1.00 mg for at least nine years, she had become virtually incapacitated by her asthma and allergies: she could no longer walk further than across the farmyard without acute dyspnoea, enter the stables or go close to the horses, or clip poodles, which was once her profession.

She woke at 3 a.m. each morning with asthma, was chilly like an icebox, perspired profusely and felt very weak.

Most of the consultation time was spent in obtaining her history. Among her formidable list of symptoms, I bypassed her infertility and gave priority to her asthma and allergies.

Examination

She was a short, overweight woman, slightly cushingoid with facial hair.

Treatment

A 30c potency of cat, dog and horse hair, mixed feathers and house dust all mixed into one preparation, weekly.

Aconite 30c quarter-hourly at onset of asthma attacks if distress and palpitations excessive.

Cuprum metallicum 30c when necessary: indicated for asthma attacks at 3 am and for cramps.

Dexamethasone 30c alternate days, hopefully to minimise further side effects from her routine medication with DM.

No change in conventional medication.

Subsequent consultations were with her husband, mainly by telephone as they lived so far away.

Progress

24.2.93. Asthma and cramps 25% improved. Still waking at 3 a.m. but not with asthma. She wanted something to ease her attacks of diarrhoea and colic and frequent tempers (large sustained doses of steroids can affect the psyche). Most significant of all, the hospital reported that her blood 17-OH had dropped from 16 to 7.8 nmol/l, which was unprecedented in the last nine years (apart from one occasion, when in error she had taken an excess of DM and been oversuppressed). My prescription was:

Reduce *Dexamethasone* 30c to two doses a week.
Kali carbonicum 30c twice daily, alternate days.
Colocynth 30c quarter-hourly for colic (*Magnesia phosphorica* 30c if *Colocynth* ineffective).
Nux vomica 30c as required for tempers.

7.3.93. 17OH = 1.60 nmol/l, lowest level ever recorded for her. DM reduced to 0.5 mg daily in case she is now oversuppressed. Repeated request for specific homeopathic treatment for infertility.

The word infertility does not appear in Kent's *Repertory* but sterility does. However, I ignored the rubric, still feeling her constitutional medicine was *Kali carb.*, and also prescribed:

Folliculinum 30c for five days, followed by *Oophorinum* 30c for five days. Ideally one or the other should be given on days 10 to 14 of the menstrual cycle (see Hunton, M. *Brit Hom J* 1993; 92:96) but she had not had a period in the last nine months.

13.3.93. 'Asthma marvellous. She has been grooming horses this week without bronchospasm for first time in nine months. Not needed nebuliser recently, salbutamol inhaler occasionally.'

2.4.93. 17-OH fallen to 0.7 nmol/l, hospital mystified.

'Could the *Dexamethasone* 30c on alternate days be affecting the blood test?' I insisted she stopped taking the remedy, to see if the 17-OH level would rise again. Such a low level of 17-OH suggests she had been grossly oversuppressed by an excess dose of steroids, yet if *Dexamethasone* 30c was interfering with the test, and making it unreliable, she could be having too little steroid and be heading for a crisis.

6.4.93. Crisis following attack of diarrhoea. No significant improvement after 100 mg IM hydrocortisone twice. She managed to stay at home, with the support of her GP. Dose of DM increased to 10 mg daily, then reduced gradually to 1 mg daily for a month without any *Dexamethasone* 30c.

15.5.93. Calm and enjoying life – she had never felt so well. Been hedging and helping in the fields. A week ago reduced daily DM from 1.0 to 0.75 mg.

She wanted to resume isopathic *Dexamethasone* 30c and wanted protection from allergy to trees and grasses; and from frequent attacks of painless diarrhoea.

Treatment

Reduce *Kali carb.* 30c from daily to every 72 hours.
Dexamethasone 30c weekly.
B2 30c and *B3* 30c grass and tree pollens, daily during season.*
Phosphoric acid 30c four times a day for diarrhoea; if ineffective try *China* 30c.
Continue DM 0.5 mg daily.

14.6.93. While she was grooming a stallion, it spun round, knocked her down, and then calmly placed a foot on her thigh, pinning her to the ground. The stallion was 17 hands, i.e. 1.83 m (6 ft) tall to its neck, and weighed a ton. Her husband quickly released her, and within a minute started giving her *Aconite* 30c. Amazingly the shock did not send her into a crisis, which it would certainly have done before she started homeopathic treatment.

She then took some *Arnica,* and later was able to walk the stallion round the ring!

Phosphoric acid did not help her diarrhoea but *China* did, seeming to work wonders.

18.9.93. Her husband reported that her asthma was still marvellous; she had been milking a mare and bottle-feeding its non-suckling foal every two hours by day and every four hours by night for three weeks, in the stable among the straw and wood shavings. In the past, close contact with a horse precipitated an asthma attack.

She had stopped taking all routine homeopathic medicines except *Dexamethasone* 30c once a week and only 0.5 mg DM daily for the last three months. She had been referred to an obstetrician for treatment for her anovulatory infertility.

---

*Isopathic allergen preparations containing the following constituents:

B2: Grass pollens – bent, brome, cocksfoot, crested dogstail, oat grass, meadow fescue, meadow foxtail, rye grass, timothy, sweet vernal, Yorkshire fog.

B3: Tree pollens – alder, ash, beech, silver birch, elm, hazel, oak, plane, poplar, willow.

29.9.93. 17-OH 5nmol/1. She was feeling very well, the fittest for years. Able to do a full day's housework; up at 4 a.m. if preparing for a distant horse show. Working in the stables and fields without total exhaustion and breathlessness, even up to 11 p.m. Clipping poodles without needing her nebuliser prophylactically; only reaction is occasional minimal chest tightness.

7.10.93. 17-OH 2nmol/1. Started on human menopausal gonadotrophin injections to promote ovulation; to be followed by daily injections of progesterone when a large enough follicle is fertilised. Consequently the 17-OH test could well be compromised. Happily she could tell immediately if her CAH was out of order and whether she was having the right maintenance dose of steroids.

20.10.93. Despite travelling a 150-mile round trip to hospital three times a week for scans to monitor the enlarging follicles, with all the excitement and stress involved, she has had no asthma or CAH upset.

28.4.94. Very much improved; asthma well controlled despite her spending much of each day grooming, harnessing and driving shire horses and preparing them for shows. Still on fertility treatment and reduced maintenance dose of DM. Taking *Dexamethasone* 30c weekly.

On 22.8.95 she had twins delivered by caesarean section at 28 weeks gestation: a boy weighing 1.3 kg (2 lb 14 oz) who subsequently died, and a girl weighing 0.68 kg (1 lb 7 oz) who is alive and well.

On 8.11.96 a professor of obstetrics and gynaecology personally delivered her of a 2.27 kg (5 lb) live girl. The CAH Group, having researched the world medical literature, have not found another recorded case of a CAH sufferer giving birth to a living baby.

September 99. Both girls continue to thrive. They do not have CAH but are carriers. The mother, now 39 years old, has a very energetic active life, looking after her young children, one of whom suffers from night terrors and wakes screaming every night. Her husband's work involves him being away from home four days and nights each week. Despite this she runs the farm and home single-handed, looking after a large farmhouse, many shire horses and ponies, sheep, dogs and other livestock.

She still takes daily prednisolone and occasionally needs conventional medication for her infrequent asthma attacks. She still obtains great benefit from homeopathic medicines, both for herself and her daughters.

ANOREXIA, ALLERGY OR ARSENIC?

CASE 127

This strange case is that of a 34-year-old woman who consulted me for gross loss of weight and weakness, constipation, and severe attacks of abdominal pain which had become worse since a cystectomy two years previously.

Her past medical history was involved. She had been constipated, taking laxatives nearly all her life, and had had frequent attacks of dyspepsia with abdominal colic. In her teens she was treated in hospital by a psychiatrist for anorexia nervosa, and made a full recovery.

In her early married life she was treated for psychosexual problems. Despite this, and fifteen years amenorrhoea, she had two children born by caesarean section, after pregnancies which necessitated prolonged bed-rest and intravenous infusions to prevent her uterus contracting. She attributed the beginning of her weight loss, after marriage, to the side effects of various fertility drugs, which resulted in pain and flooding, hospital admissions, and finally hysterectomy.

After this she began to suffer from dysuria and frequency (160 times in 24 hours), was readmitted to hospital many times, and ultimately referred to the professor of neurosurgery.

An autonomic block was performed but was only effective for a short time, and finally she had a total cystectomy with ileal conduit. The histology of the bladder showed gross fibromuscular thickening with inflammatory infiltration, but no cancer or TB. She made a satisfactory post-operative recovery, but still complained bitterly of pain in the left iliac fossa, and constipation. She lost weight after the operation, in spite of an apparently normal diet. She then had a pulmonary embolism, and was put on an anticoagulant.

During the next year she was admitted to a different Midlands teaching hospital, before being transferred by ambulance to a London hospital that specialised in diseases of the rectum and colon. A psychiatrist and a neurologist were of the opinion that she had major psychological problems, but that there was also a physical basis for her symptoms. Her pain was treated with analgesics, her constipation with enemas, and later with magnesium sulphate crystals. A nasogastric tube feed of about 2000 calories daily resulted in a weight gain of almost 3 kg (6.6 lb), but had to be discontinued because she developed an upper respiratory infection and complained of nausea when the tube feed was restarted.

As she continued to decline, and her weight had reverted to 31.8 kg

(70 lb), she was told frankly that she should be admitted to a psychiatric ward. She resented and declined this advice, and ultimately, in desperation, sought homeopathic treatment.

7.11.83. Her husband brought her by car, as she was too weak to drive herself.

Her symptoms were :

1) Weight loss – weight 31.8 kg (70 lb), had been 46 kg (101 lb) until three years ago.
2) Depression. Neither she nor her husband expected her to live until Christmas.
3) Weakness and exhaustion.
4) Feeling very cold. Occasionally, head hot and sweaty, body icy cold.
5) Mental restlessness.
6) Fastidious. 'Dreadfully so. I have to be organised.'
7) Thirst, unquenchable for hot drinks.
8) Ravenous appetite, eating voraciously – including half a pound of chocolate daily to gain weight, 'yet I am steadily losing weight'. Often eating bread and butter and biscuits at midnight, and again at 3 a.m.
9) Craving for meat fat ('I eat all the fat off the plates at meal-times'), and for cheese and cream. No craving for salt.
10) Terrible indigestion.
11) Constipation 'unless I take the Epsom salts five times a day that the hospital prescribed.'
12) Worse until 10 a.m.
13) Worse for thunder.
14) Easy bruising.

She was on a high fibre diet, and smoked thirty cigarettes daily.

Medication: As well as the magnesium sulphate crystals, she was on painkillers and antispasmodic drugs prescribed by the hospital and her GP.

Treatment

Arsenicum album seemed clearly indicated, as it covered the mental restlessness, coldness, weakness, the midnight aggravation of hunger, the craving for fat and thirst for hot drinks. I gave her *Arsenicum album* 10M, one dose to be taken at once, and *Calcarea phosphorica* 3c, to be taken four times daily. Also *Colocynth* 30c as required for severe colic.

I instructed her to continue taking any conventional medicine which was being prescribed, i.e. Epsom Salts, as homeopathic treatment, in general, is additional to conventional treatment.

Doubting the veracity of her account of her medical history, I contacted her GP, who allowed me unrestrained access to her medical records and hospital reports, and confirmed her statement that in the previous twelve years she had spent a total of five years as an inpatient in teaching hospitals, at no time being in a psychiatric ward.

Five weeks later she was much improved, having stopped all analgesics after four days. She still had violent attacks of colic, which were relieved by *Colocynth*. She stopped drinking whole milk, substituting skimmed milk. She replaced the Epsom Salts with a herbal laxative, and took *Nux vomica* 30c for dyspepsia. At this point she received another single dose of *Arsenicum alb.* 10M and *Cuprum met.* 30c when necessary for cramps, and *Calc. phos.* 3c was discontinued.

Improvement and weight gain continued, and two months later she was demonstrated at a homeopathic doctors' meeting at Selly Oak Hospital, where it was suggested that she was suffering from an allergy to milk, because of her craving for milk, cream and cheese, all of which upset her, and because of a typical history. She was advised to avoid all cow and goat milk products, and to take *Lac vaccinum* 30c weekly.

Her health continued to improve, although she remained allergic to milk products, and when she had regained her former weight of 46 kg (101 lb) she and her husband held a dinner party to celebrate the fact. The guests included the doctors and specialists who had helped her.

Discussion

The cause for her bladder becoming fibrosed and shrunken may never be established. Her continued loss of weight and abdominal pain could have been psychogenic in origin, and one psychiatrist felt she was suffering from a relapse of teenage anorexia nervosa.

The patient insisted that she only restricted her eating at that time because of the colic she experienced after most meals. It could be postulated, in support of a psychogenic aetiology, that she responded at last to a sympathetic listener who accepted her story, and believed her symptoms were mainly organic. She felt that such was the case, and it resulted in her deciding to fight problems to which she had already succumbed.

A more probable alternative diagnosis is that of a masked milk allergy, and withholding milk was followed by a remarkable improvement in her health. In this condition the patient craves for, and depends on, the very foods he or she has become allergic to.

In support of this diagnosis :

- Her father never drank milk or took it in tea or coffee. She never knew why.
- When a baby she screamed so much that her mother had to send her away for two weeks' respite. All her milk teeth were black on eruption, and were removed.
- Her own daughter suffered from eczema, and was very allergic to milk.
- Her son was allergic to orange and fish fingers. He craved both, but became very emotionally disturbed after eating either of them.
- No one had ever asked her about food allergies; she had mainly been in surgical, gynaecological or orthopaedic wards.

Mackarness, a recognised authority on this subject, says in his book *Not All in the Mind*:

Masking is characteristic of stage two of the specific adaptation syndrome, when the subject is adapting well ... But ... the stages of adaptation are a continuum, ending in stage three, towards which the victim is moving inexorably. As stage three is entered, there is exhaustion of the hormonal and enzyme resources needed to remain normal in the face of stress exerted by a particular allergenic food. Now every meal brings, not a temporary pick-up, but a devastating onset of symptoms.

This patient would appear to have reached this stage in her illness, and most of the symptoms she had been treated for are prominent in his list of criteria for suspecting food allergy. If this is so, a remark she once made in hospital assumes a new relevance: 'The only time I begin to feel well in hospital is after an operation, when I am on a drip (intravenous infusion) and do not have to eat anything. I sometimes wish I could be on a permanent drip.' Admittedly a psychiatrist and an ecologist would deduct different conclusions from that statement.

What is most interesting is that her dramatic improvement began within a few days of taking the first dose of *Arsenicum album* 10M, at least two weeks before she substituted skimmed for whole milk in her diet. At that time neither she nor I knew anything about masked allergy. She attributed the improvement to my having restored her hope. She may have been right, or was it the *Arsenicum* whose provings matched her symptoms so closely? *Post hoc ergo propter hoc.*

The account ends where it began. The question marks remain. Was it anorexia, was it allergy, was it *Arsenicum*, or was it all three ?

TERMINAL ILLNESS

Arsenicum album has long had the reputation of calming the mental and physical restlessness of death throes. Some have claimed that used in high potency it acts as euthanasia, but I doubt this; I have used it for fifty years in the last stages of terminal illness, and only on one occasion did I have cause to wonder.

CASE 128

Many years ago I was called in the early evening to a man who was obviously dying and was very distressed, as were all the assembled family. I offered to administer some medicine that would ease him. I explained that what I was about to give would not in any way act like euthanasia, but it should help to calm his mental anguish. I then asked for a glass of warm water, stirred into it about a dozen grains of *Arsenicum alb.* 10M, and instructed the relatives to give the patient a teaspoon dose every quarter hour, until I called again some hours later. This medication would also involve the relatives, who felt they were helpless in this situation. I intended returning about three hours later, and was surprised to get a message about three-quarters of an hour later to say the patient was dead.

On returning, I detected a certain unusual restraint in the room, and with every eye watching me, a spokesman asked, 'And what shall we do with the remaining medicine, doctor?'

Realising that this was a loaded question, and that they suspected me of having used euthanasia after all, I replied, 'Pour it down the sink', and then as an afterthought, 'Or you could drink it.' I then picked up the glass and drained the contents! After that the tense atmosphere lifted. The patient had apparently died quite peacefully.

Years later I recounted this event at a seminar on homeopathy. In the question time that followed the lecture a doctor chided me facetiously for being so rash as to drink the water. On asking him why, he replied, 'Because, after you left, someone might have added real arsenic to it!'

CASE 129

A doctor in his mid-fifties was critically ill with methotrexate poisoning. He was grossly overweight and diabetic, and had been virtually bedfast for the last eight months. Recently he had become jaundiced, and developed ascites and oedema, with pyrexia and confusion.

Two consultants had visited him and diagnosed 'liver failure and encephalopathy', and advised discontinuing all medication. He had had a marked antipathy to homeopathy all his life, and was very prejudiced against it, but in a lucid interval had given way to his wife, who insisted that he should try it.

I was not able to visit him for two days, but was told of the following symptoms:

He was very restless and had to be helped change his position every ten minutes, day and night. He kept trying to get out of bed, but was too weak.

He suffered from intense burning paraesthesia of the skin all over his body.

Despite this:

He was very cold, needing the room temperature at about 27°C (80°F).

He felt nauseated, complained of a burning heat in his stomach, and requested frequent sips of warm water, which he promptly vomited back.

His set of symptoms so exactly matched those produced by arsenical poisoning, that I advised giving him *Arsenicum album* 30c in warm water every quarter of an hour until relief of his symptoms.

Thirty-six hours later I visited him to find the house full of relatives, many of them doctors.

The patient was lying, apparently at ease, smiling and able to greet me. His wife was full of gratitude.

Following taking *Arsenicum album* in water:

He had had his first night's sleep for weeks, and had had no further melaena, nor the usual need to open his bowels two or three times each night.

All the burning paraesthesia of the skin had subsided. 'Look,' his wife said, 'he can let me touch his legs and pull his socks on. He would not let me do that before.'

The oedema of his ankles had disappeared, and the abdomen was no longer so tense, though the skin was still stretched and shiny.

His burning gastralgia had settled, and he was retaining fluids.

His mind and memory were now clear, with no delusional thoughts.

What was surprising was that the ascites and oedema had significantly improved, despite frusemide being discontinued after his first dose of *Arsenicum.*

A week later his improvement was still maintained, but he now had developed:

- More bruises and purpuric spots
- Photophobia
- A craving for ice-cold water
- Uncontrolled glycosuria, despite having started insulin therapy again.

On these indications, the prescription was changed to *Phosphorus* 30c every four hours.

Four days later he was admitted urgently to hospital with severe abdominal pain, which was diagnosed as an acute gastric ulcer. He developed renal suppression, and his output of urine fell to 70ml/24 hours for three days. He was given *Apis* 30c every two hours, and his output rose again.

Four days later he was given *Eel serum* 30c at two-hourly intervals, as this has the reputation of lowering the blood urea in uraemia.

Several weeks later, and having had a blood transfusion, he was able to return home. His condition deteriorated steadily, but he appeared to benefit from regular doses of *Arsenicum.* The night before he died he became increasingly restless again, but each time *Arsenicum album* 10M was given it temporarily calmed him, and relieved the intense burning sensation in his stomach.

This history illustrates:

- The use of homeopathic medicine even in advanced incurable illness. It can improve the quality of life, and help ease the distress of dying.
- The need to change the medicines as the symptoms change.
- The use of animal medicines (honey bee and eel). Had the melaena increased, I would have prescribed *Crotalus horridus* (rattlesnake) which is indicated in septicaemia with multiple haemorrhages (and in yellow fever).
- That homeopathic medicine can be given concurrently with conventional medicines, and still prove effective.
- That homeopathy works even when the patient is unaware that he is being treated by it, or is unconscious. This establishes that it does not work by means of suggestion.

CONCLUSION

The cases reported in this book have been collected over a lifetime of medical practice, and have been meticulously recorded. Many tell of remarkable improvements, although in themselves do not prove anything – but they do add to the growing body of evidence that homeopathy is an effective therapeutic method.

In the past, collections of cases such as these have been subject to ridicule as purely anecdotal. However, in this day of evidence-based medicine, it is now recognised that measures of patient satisfaction are indeed valid criteria against which to judge a system of therapeutics.

Indeed, such a collection of cases can now be judged to be 'Anecdotal but Significant'.

Chapter 15

How Hahnemann Pre-empted Many Ideas of Modern Medicine

I feel it would be fitting to dedicate the last chapter of this book to the person whose brilliance established homeopathy as a rational form of treatment.

It is now more than 150 years since Hahnemann died, so it is an appropriate time to review and evaluate his life's work, researches and discoveries.

I have no difficulty in remembering the date of Hahnemann's death; he died in 1843, exactly one century before the year in which I qualified.

In so many ways his discoveries were far ahead of his times, and his prescience was remarkable. There will only be space to consider a few of the most significant, so the list is not exhausting.

Heroic Medicine
His methods were revolutionary. He lived in an age of heroic medicine when massive bloodletting, purging and polypharmacy were the accepted treatments both here in Europe and in America. As an example: on 14.12.1799, when Hahnemann was forty-four years old, George Washington developed a severe sore throat. His chronicler reported: 'It was inflamed and gave him some difficulty in breathing. His overseer removed a pint of blood, but it provided no relief. A physician was called, who soon after his arrival applied a blister to the throat and let another pint of blood. At three o'clock that afternoon, two other doctors came to consult with the first one, and by a vote of two to one they decided to let more blood, removing a quart that time. They reported that blood flowed 'slow and thick'. By then the President was dehydrated, and it would seem that the doctors must have had to squeeze out the final drops of blood. Washington died sometime between ten and eleven that same night (aged sixty-seven years). In his case heroic treatment consisted of the removal of at least four pints of blood, blistering and a dose of calomel. Perhaps he would have died in any case, but the treatment certainly provided no relief.

Hahnemann was revolted by such treatments and decried them vociferously. Nowadays the only vestige of bloodletting is in donating blood, in exchange transfusions, in blood disorders where the body makes too much blood and in the use of leeches to reduce bruising and haematomas in delicate microsurgery.

I was shown round a leech farm in Wales when on holiday recently, though it is now no longer open to the public. I was allowed to handle and photograph some of the thousands of leeches that they dispatch to hospitals all over the British Isles and abroad. They claim to be the world's only legal source of medicinal leeches, and recently have opened a subsidiary company in South Carolina to supply the USA and Canada.

Jenner & Hunter – Contemporaries

Hahnemann was contemporary with Edward Jenner, the British physician and pioneer of vaccinations. In 1796 Jenner found that smallpox could be prevented by inoculation with the substance from cowpox lesions. Hahnemann was also contemporary with John Hunter, the famous anatomist and surgeon, who is rightly considered to be the founder of scientific surgery.

Hunter developed angina in his mid-forties, and as it progressed he recognised that his life was 'in the hands of any rascal who chose to annoy and tease him'. When he was sixty-eight years old he was contradicted whilst speaking at a board meeting at St George's Hospital, and collapsed and died immediately. He was buried in St Martin-in-the-Fields, but in 1859 his remains were removed to Westminster Abbey.

It is on record that Jenner once asked Hunter, 'Do you think that cowpox injections could prevent smallpox?' Hunter replied, 'Try it and see.' Hahnemann bemoaned the fact that his colleagues would not test homeopathy and see if it could cure illness.

Prophylaxis

Hahnemann refers to Jenner's work in his *Organon*. In the first edition, in 1818, he wrote 'Could the cowpox protect us from smallpox otherwise than homeopathically? Without mentioning any other traits of close resemblance existing between these two maladies they have this in common: they generally appear but once during the course of a person's life; they leave behind similar deep cicatrices; they both occasion tumefaction of the axillary glands; fevers that are analogous, an inflamed areola around each pack, and an ophthalmia and convulsions.'

In later editions he interpreted his observations, and theorised:

The cowpox would cure this malady when already present if the smallpox were not stronger than it. To produce this effect then it only wants that excess of power which according to the law of nature, ought to accompany the homeopathic resemblance in order to affect a cure. We can, therefore, only employ this homeopathic remedy previous to the appearance of the stronger smallpox. When so employed it excites a disease very similar (homeopathic) to the smallpox; after it has run its course, as the human body can as a rule only be attacked once in its life with a disease of this nature (cowpox or smallpox), it is henceforward protected for life against cow or smallpox.

He called this mode of homeopathic cure an antecession (now known as prophylaxis).

Controlled Trials

A parallel example of homeopathy preceding conventional medicine is in the field of allergy and desensitisation. It is relevant to refer to the work of Dr David Reilly and his colleagues in Glasgow, whose controlled trial of a homeopathic preparation of mixed grass pollens in the treatment of hayfever was published in the *Lancet* in 1986.

This randomised double-blind placebo-controlled trial showed that the action of homeopathic medicines was more than a placebo effect. They observed: 'Blackley was an established homeopathic physician before he identified pollen as a precipitant cause of hayfever, and his now classical work was first published as a series of articles in the *British Journal of Homeopathy*.'

Homeopathic physicians were using potentised pollen-containing extracts in hayfever at least twenty years before Noon introduced injections in 1911. Coulter, a medical historian, argues that the link between immunotherapy and homeopathy is well established; he cites von Behring, one of the founders of immunotherapy, for presaging immunotherapy and serum therapy: 'von Behring thus gave an unsolicited and independent vindication of Hahnemann's system of therapy.'

A True Scientist

Hahnemann was a true scientist and challenged the accepted wisdom of his day. He questioned Cullen's theory that quinine (cinchona) suppressed marsh fever (malaria) because quinine was a powerful astringent. Being a chemist himself he knew there were far stronger astringents than quinine, but which could not control marsh fever.

He proved medicines individually on himself and other volunteers, and accurately and laboriously recorded all the side effects they experienced. He must have been one of the first to keep a log diary. But more importantly, having discovered a medical phenomenon which could not be (and still has not been) rationally explained, he did not simply dismiss it as being impossible and deny its existence, but spent the rest of his life trying to refine and develop the system.

Allergens

In recent years an impetus has been provided for using homeopathic immunotherapy to desensitise patients against the allergens to which they are allergic. This is because GPs have effectively been banned from using the standard desensitising injections in their surgeries, unless they are prepared to stay with the patient in the surgery for several hours, and have means of resuscitation in the event of the patient collapsing from an anaphylactic reaction. The medical defence societies will not otherwise cover the doctor against litigation.

Happily, in my experience, very satisfactory results follow using homeopathic oral preparations of the allergens; they appear to be as effective, if not more so, than conventional injections. This applies to numerous allergies: house dust mite, horse dander, dog hair, cat fur, feathers, grass pollens, flowers, moulds, and so on – the list increases annually.

Time Aggravations

Hahnemann also observed and recorded the time aggravation of many homeopathic medicines, especially those of mineral origin.

I first appreciated the significance of this about twelve years ago at a meeting of the Midlands Homeopathy Research Group. We had invited an eminent nephrologist, who was also a leading authority on circadian rhythms, to talk to us about his special interest in 'Circadian Variations in Conventional Medicine'. He was impressed by the list of symptoms and the time aggravations recorded for homeopathic medicines in Kent's repertory.

He had studied biorhythms for many years, and was particularly intrigued by the 2–4 a.m. time aggravation for *Kali carbonicum* (potassium carbonate). He explained that measuring blood electrolytes (sodium, potassium, etc.) at different times of the day and night revealed that a distinct change in potassium level took place at about

3 a.m. every twenty-four hours. Yet Hahnemann had stumbled across this modality without being able to explain it, at least a century earlier.

Our visiting specialist had not only discovered many cyclical variations which occurred in the body every twenty-four hours, but also some which occurred at seven day intervals; again Hahnemann had identified homeopathic medicines that had aggravations at seven and even fourteen day intervals, which we use to control illnesses with either of these features. These are listed in Kent's repertory under 'Periodic', so that, for instance, in the case of migraine occurring every weekend one would look under the section 'Head' and the sub-sections: 'pain, periodic headache, every seven days' (*Phosphorus, Silica, Sulphur, Tuberculinum*, etc.).

How astute Hahnemann and his colleagues and followers were in observing and recording these time factors of the medicines they proved.

A Century Ahead of his Time

There are many imponderables in homeopathy. For instance, what prescience led our homeopathic forbears to use vanadium, which would only later be discovered to be an oxygen carrier and hence therapeutic in wasting diseases? Boericke advised using the 6–12c potency in wasting diseases on that account.

Hahnemann was also a century ahead of his time in the treatment of mental illness, which in his day was barbaric. Space precludes elaborating on his humane methods of treatment. He was also in advance of his day in his views on hygiene, housing and diet, and most interestingly, hypnosis.

He applauded the correct use of hypnosis, which in his day was called 'animal magnetism' or 'Mesmerism', and which was proscribed by the medical profession. He wrote: 'This curative force, often so stupidly denied and disdained for a century, is a marvellous priceless gift of God to mankind, by means of which the strong will of a well-intentioned person upon a sick one ... can bring the vital energy of the healthy mesmeriser endowed with this power into another person dynamically (just as one of the poles of a powerful magnetic rod upon a bar of steel).' (*Organon* 6th edition)

Hypnosis

Admittedly he accepted the erroneous view of his day as to how hypnosis worked, but then he died in 1843, the very year in which the Scottish doctor Braid published his book on hypnosis. In this Braid dismissed all supernatural and 'magnetic' powers and forces. By means of careful and controlled experiments, he was able to ascribe all the phenomena to a change in the state of the nervous system of the subject, which he called 'nervous sleep', or 'neurypnology'.

Today we regard hypnosis as a state of altered attention. Hahnemann, though limited in his understanding of the mechanism of hypnosis (as with homeopathy), at least welcomed it when he had seen dramatic cures resulting from its use.

In summary, when we consider his prescience in all these aspects of medical theory and treatment, we have to acknowledge his brilliance. Hahnemann was a genius whose name and honour deserve to be perpetuated.

Home Remedy Kit

Useful homeopathic home remedies for acute conditions. These are generally available from retail outlets in the 6c potency. I find that the 30c potency will work to better effect when sufficient of the indications listed below for a particular remedy are present.

ACONITE: SHOCK and No. 1 FEVER
For shock, croup, effects of fright or chills; any emergency, e.g. accident, animal bites, asthma, haemorrhage, bereavement (if fear), distress, breathlessness, palpitations, tremblings, or numb feelings. At onset of fevers, if thirsty, restless, anxious.

Dose: 10 granules (one tablet or pill) every 15 minutes until relief.

ANTIMONIUM CRUDUM: No. 2 STOMACH
When cross, touchy, depressed. Vomits feeds, white-coated tongue, corners of mouth cracked. No appetite. Sick headaches from catarrh, alcohol, bathing. Wants sharp drinks, or pickles. Belching, bloating.

Dose: 10 granules (one tablet or pill) every 15 minutes until relief.

ANTIMONIUM TARTARICUM: No. 2 COUGH
When touchy, drowsy, very weak. Cold clammy sweat; pale or bluish face, white-coated tongue. Breathless, suffocating, gasping; must sit up. Rattling cough, unable to expectorate. Worse warmth.

Dose: 10 granules (one tablet or pill) every 15 minutes until relief.

ARNICA: INJURY
For bruises, sprains, concussion, crushed fingers, road accidents, etc. If shocked, give *Aconite* first. Also for exhaustion, or muscle aching (heart, chest, back or limbs) from strain, sport, or overuse. Use before and after dental surgery.

Dose: 10 granules (one tablet or pill) every 2 hours until relief.

ARSENICUM ALBUM: SICKNESS and DIARRHOEA
When sickness and diarrhoea simultaneously (?gastric flu, ?food poisoning), feeling very cold, anxious, exhausted, can't rest. Burning pains in stomach. Thirst for warm drinks. Can't bear sight, smell of food.

Dose: 10 granules, every 15 minutes until relief.

BELLADONNA: EARACHE and No. 2 FEVER
When burning hot, flushed, wide-eyed, excited, ?delirious (?scarlet rash). Thirsty but won't drink. Also sore throats, colic, throbbing headaches, throbbing boils, severe earache with the above symptoms. Effects of sunstroke.

Dose: 10 granules (one tablet or pill) every 15 minutes until relief.

BRYONIA: PAIN and HEADACHE
For bursting headaches, migraine, arthritis, pleurisy, only when pains are worse from movement, breathing, warmth; better for pressure, lying quiet, keeping still in cool. Irritable, parched, thirst for cold drinks.

Dose: 10 granules (one tablet or pill) every 4 hours until relief.

CAMPHOR: CHILL
When icy cold following chill. First stage of a cold, when chilled, sneezing, better warmth. Onset of diarrhoea from chill, if feeling 'frozen'.

Dose: 10 granules (one tablet or pill) every 5 minutes, until relief and feeling warm. Keep bottle separate. Camphor vapour inactivates other homeopathic medicines.

CANTHARIS: BLADDER and BURNS
Cystitis when urine scalds, passed drop by drop. Unbearable urging and frequency. Also burns and scalds, better for cold applications. Also burning, itching blisters (erysipelas). Insect bites.

Dose: 10 granules (one tablet or pill) every 2 hours until relief.

CARBO VEGETABILIS: WIND and COLLAPSE
When stomach distended, passing wind up (?and down), must sit up, loosen clothing. When collapsed, ?pale, ?bluish, cold, cold sweat, needs propping up, gasping, must have air and be fanned.

Dose: 10 granules (one tablet or pill) every 15 minutes until relief.

227

CHAMOMILLA: FRANTIC PAIN

For unbearable pain; earache, toothache, teething, better being picked up, ?one cheek hot. Colic, diarrhoea, green motions. Bad tempered, impatient, worse heat, anger.

Dose: 10 granules every 5 minutes until relief.

COLOCYNTH: COLIC

For agonising colic, better doubling up, hard pressure, heat, twisting about. Griping pains causing distension, belching, vomiting, ?diarrhoea. Colic and neuralgia from anger or 'getting worked up'.

Dose: 10 granules (one tablet or pill) every 15 minutes until relief.

EUPHRASIA: HAYFEVER and No. 1 MEASLES

For onset of measles when eyes streaming, tears burn, can't face light. Running nose, sneezing, cough. Throbbing headache. Hayfever, as above, worse indoors warmth, evenings.

Dose: 10 granules (one tablet or pill) every 15 minutes until relief.

GELSEMIUM: INFLUENZA and 'NERVES'

When hot, flushed, aching, trembling, dizzy, drowsy, feeling 'drugged' or weak. Headache, limbs and eyes feel heavy, back chilly. Sneezing, running nose. Sore throat, difficulty swallowing. No thirst. Also, upsets from 'nerves'.

Dose: 10 granules (one tablet or pill) every 2 hours until relief.

IPECACUANHA: NAUSEA and No. 1 COUGH

For persistent nausea, ?vomiting, with clean tongue, much saliva. Onset violent, suffocating, wheezing bouts, coughing. Also nose bleeds, haemorrhages, with nausea.

Dose: 10 granules (one tablet or pill) every 2 hours until relief.

MERCURIUS SOLUBILIS: FEVERISH COLD

When feeling chilly in cold, hot in warmth, weak, trembling, offensive sweat and breath. Profuse greenish catarrh, salivation, thirst. Diarrhoea with persistent straining, slime, ?blood. All symptoms worse at night.

Dose: 10 granules (one tablet or pill) every 2 hours until relief.

NATRUM MURIATICUM: RECURRENT COLD and DEPRESSION

For sneezy colds with cold sores, if much nasal catarrh; if feeling cold, but worse in warm room. Greasy skin, likes salt, thirsty. Also depression, if irritable, weary, ?weepy (but on doctor's advice only).

Dose: 10 granules (one tablet or pill) every 4 hours until relief.

NUX VOMICA: STOMACH and No. 2 FLU
When chilly, irritable, quarrelsome. Delayed indigestion, nausea, constipation, or frequent unsatisfactory bowel actions. Itching piles. Flu or raw throat, if chilled when uncovered. Stuffy colds if worse in cold air. Infant's snuffles, if irritable.

Dose: 10 granules (one tablet or pill) every 4 hours until relief.

PHOSPHORUS: LARYNGITIS and REPEATED VOMITING
When chest tight, hoarse, hurts to talk, ?loss of voice. Dry, tickling cough, worse cold air, worse talking. Gastritis with craving for cold drinks, often vomited immediately. Nervous. Thunder headaches.

Dose: 10 granules (one tablet or pill) every 2 hours until relief.

PULSATILLA: CATARRH and No. 2 MEASLES
When thick, coloured catarrh, of eyelids or nose. Loss of smell. Dry mouth (no thirst). Better in open air. Catarrhal cough, worse in warm room. measles. Indigestion from fat, rich food.

Dose: 10 granules (one tablet or pill) every 4 hours until relief.

RHUS TOXICODENDRON: RHEUMATISM and ARTHRITIS
When pains, stiffness, worse in wet weather, cold air, in bed, after rest (first movements hurt). Better keeping moving. Flu, dry cough with the above symptoms. Also itching blisters (?erysipelas, ?shingles) if restless. Tendon sprains.

Dose: 10 granules (one tablet or pill) every 4 hours until relief.

SULPHUR: RASHES
For burning, itching skin rashes, worse for warmth, worse from scratching, washing, clothing. Burning boils, styes and piles. Hungry, easily fatigued, hot flushes, hot feet (uncovers them in bed). Morning diarrhoea.

Dose: 10 granules (one tablet or pill) twice daily until relief. Maximum 6 doses.

Bibliography

Boericke, W. & O. *Pocket Manual of Homoeopathic Materia Medica*, 9th ed. 1927

Clarke, J.H. *Dictionary of Practical Materia Medica* 1900-2

Collier, J.A.B., Longmore, J.M., Harvey, J.H. *Oxford Handbook of Clinical Specialties*, 3rd ed. 1991:222

Congenital Adrenal Hyperplasia, National Organization for Rare Diseases, New Fairfield, Connecticut, USA

Culpeper, N. *Complete Herbal and English Physician* 1652

Gibson Miller, R. *Relationship of Remedies* 1933

Hahnemann, S. *The Chronic Diseases. Their peculiar nature and their homoeopathic cure* trans. L.H. Tafel 1896

Hahnemann, S. *Materia Medica Pura* trans. R.E. Dudgeon 1880

Hahnemann, S. *Organon of Medicine* (5th and 6th editions) trans. R.E. Dudgeon & W. Boericke 1922

Hering, C. *Condensed Materia Medica*, 4th ed. 1894

Hughes, R. *A Manual of Pharmacodynamics,* 5th ed. 1886; 7th ed. 1931

Hunton, M. 'Endometriosis and homoeopathy' *Br Hom J* 1993;92:96

Hunton, M. 'Homoeopathy in the treatment of haemophilia' *Br Hom J* 1991; 80:82

Jack, R.A.F. 'How I treat Crohn's disease' *Br Hom J* 1993;82:29-36

Kent, J.T. *Lectures on Homoeopathic Materia Medica*, 1st ed. 1911; 4th ed. 1932

Kent, J.T. *Repertory of the Homoeopathic Materia Medica* , 1st ed. 1898; 6th ed. 1957

Kleijnen, J. et al. 'Clinical trials of homoeopathy' *BMJ* 1991;302:316-33

Lilienthal, S. *Homoeopathic Therapeutics*, 3rd ed. 1890

Mackarness, R. *Not All in the Mind* 1976

McLeod, J.G. 'Peripheral neuropathy' *Medicine* 1980;34:1756

Nash, E.B. *Leaders in Homoeopathic Therapeutics* 1926

Bibliography

Paterson, J. 'The Bowel Nosodes' *Br Hom J* 1950;40

Reik, T. *Psychology of Sex Relations* 1945; Pan 1961:218

Reilly, D. et al. 'Is homoeopathy a placebo response? Controlled trial of homoeopathic potency, with pollen in hayfever as model' *Lancet* 1986;ii:881-6

Tyler, M.L. *Homoeopathic Drug Pictures*, 1st ed. 1942; 2nd ed. 1952

Tyler, M.L. *Pointers to the Common Remedies* (Nos. 1-9) British Homeopathic Association 1934

Abbreviations

ACE inhibitor angiotension-converting enzyme
BCG   Bacillus Calmette-Guérin (antituberculosis vaccine)
BMJ   *British Medical Journal*
BP   blood pressure
CAT   computerised axial tomometry (3-dimensional X-ray)
CNS   central nervous system
CSF   cerebrospinal fluid
EEG   electro-encephalogram (recording of brain-waves)
ENT   ear, nose and throat
ESR   erythrocyte sedimentation rate (blood test showing degree of
         inflammation in body)
ME   myalgic encephalomyelitis
MRI   magnetic resonance imaging
PEF   peak expiratory flow (a measure of lung capacity)
PMT   premenstrual tension
PUO   pyrexia of unknown origin
RA   rheumatoid arthritis
sac lac placebo tablets of lactose
TS   tuberous sclerosis

Remedy Index

233

Chelidonium, 50
Chenopodium anthelminticum, 47, 48, 49, 50
Chimaphila umbellata, 156
China, 38, 49, 133, 158, 210
Chininum arsenicosum, 49
Chininum sulphuricum, 48, 50
Chlorum, 83
Cicuta virosa, 44, 46, 50
Cimicifuga, 148, 172
Cina, 36, 39
Cinchona, 222
Cistus canadensis, 175
Clematis erecta, 156
Cocculus, 32, 48, 58, 59, 63, 124, 125
Coccus cacti, 15, 93
Coffea, 49
Conium, 49, 50, 156, 158, 159
Convallaria, 109
Crataegus, 9, 109
Crocus sativa, 15, 154
Crotalus horridus, 38, 218
Cuprum metallicum, 64, 123, 124, 133, 176, 208, 214

Dexamethasone, 208, 209, 210, 211
Dulcamara, 183
Dysenteriae co., 131

Echinacea, 84
Eel serum, 218
Equisetum, 65, 66, 67, 156, 157
Eupatorium perfoliatum, 205
Euphrasia, 5, 75, 76, 78, 228

Ferrum phosphoricum, 21
Ferrum picricum, 155, 156
Fluoric acid, 15, 17
Folliculinum, 209

Gaertner, 131
Gambogia, 132, 134
Gelsemium, 38, 201, 228
Glonoine, 30
Graphites, 50, 192, 193
Grass pollens, 210
Gratiola, 15, 154

Hamamelis, 14, 15, 112, 158

Hecla lava, 173, 174
Helleborus, 28
Helonias, 154
Hepar sulphuris, 21, 57, 133, 196, 197
Horse dander, 81,
House dust, 91, 99, 100
House dust mite, 81
Hyoscyamus, 13, 37, 38, 39, 41, 42
Hypercal, 27, 29
Hypericum, 27

Iberis, 110, 112
Ignatia, 32
Iodum, 15, 16, 126, 129, 141, 156
Ipecacuanha, 3, 32, 116, 117, 120, 228

Kali bichromicum, 95, 100
Kali bromatum, 196
Kali carbonicum, 38, 49, 98, 209, 210, 223
Kali iodatum, 15, 141
Kali phosphoricum, 202
Kali sulphuricum, 15, 16
Kalmia, 50

Lac vaccinum, 214
Lachesis, 15, 32, 33, 72, 141, 144, 146, 152, 154, 166, 196, 198
Lathyrus, 60, 176
Ledum palustre, 15, 27, 29, 164, 165, 166, 167, 168, 182
Lilium tigrinum, 15, 154
Lime, 79
Lycopodium, 9, 15, 38, 90, 105, 106, 108, 129, 131, 139, 140, 146, 158, 159, 160, 161, 162
Lycopus virginicus, 110, 111

Magnesia phosphorica, 57, 139, 140, 209
Manganum, 38
Medorrhinum, 88, 158, 169, 180, 182
Melilotus, 97
Menyanthes, 60
Mephitis, 93
Mercurius solubilis, 141, 183, 200, 228
Mezereum, 57
Millefolium, 97

General Index

237

– NOTES –

– NOTES –

CLASSICAL HOMOEOPATHY

Dr Margery Blackie (ed. Dr Charles Elliott & Dr Frank Johnson), 363pp, 216x138mm, 1986, with repertory, 0906584140

Draws into one volume Dr Blackie's teaching over the whole span of her career, setting before the reader the enthusiasm, learning and deep clinical understanding of one of the foremost homoeopaths of our time.

COMPARATIVE MATERIA MEDICA

Dr Eugenio F. Candegabe, 330pp, 216x138mm, 1997, 0906584361

In this comparative study of thirty-seven remedies, Dr Candegabe displays how the materia medica may be reconstructed through the mental symptoms of the repertory, so as to find the remedy whose action most closely corresponds to the dynamic totality of an individual patient's life.

EVERYDAY HOMOEOPATHY, 2nd Edition

Dr David Gemmell, 225pp, 210x148mm, 1997, 0906584442

A successful handbook for the use of homoeopathy in the everyday context of one's personal and family health care. Covers 116 problems that a lay person is quite likely to encounter and have to cope with, either as first aid or else in a wide variety of complaints and disorders which may not be urgent but where relief and cure are sought.

HOMOEOPATHIC PRESCRIBING

Dr Noel Pratt, 87pp plus 78pp interleaved, 216x120mm, revised edition 1985, 0906584035

Written for all who use homoeopathic remedies. One hundred and fifty-six common complaints and disorders are covered. Clear indications are given wherever it is important that the lay person should also obtain medical advice.

HOMOEOPATHIC TREATMENT OF BEEF AND DAIRY CATTLE

Christopher Day, MRCVS, VetFFHom, 141pp, 216x138mm, 1995, 090658437X

Written for the farmer and smallholder who wishes to use homoeopathy in the treatment of their cattle, both as individual animals and in a group. It is also of relevance to homoeopaths more generally, as it casts valuable light on ways of assessing a condition homoeopathically.

HOMOEOPATHIC TREATMENT OF ECZEMA

Robin Logan, RSHom, 152pp, 216x138mm, 1998, 0906584477

Eczema is one of the most commonly encountered conditions in everyday practice and can pose difficult and perplexing problems for the homoeopath. This book sets out a practical basis for its treatment within the context of classical homoeopathy.

HOMOEOPATHY

Dr Tomás Pablo Paschero, ed. Dr Patricia Haas, 257pp, 216x138mm, 2000, 0906584418

Dr Paschero was a classical homoeopath of the pure Kentian school – he trained with Kent's immediate successor, Dr Grimmer. The book demonstrates a deep level of insight and understanding of the classical method.

HOMOEOPATHY AS ART AND SCIENCE

Dr Elizabeth Wright Hubbard (ed. Dr Maesimund Panos & Della DesRosiers), 344pp, 216x138mm, 1990, 0906584264

This book represents a large part of Dr Hubbard's teaching writing, and conveys her great gift of being able to describe homoeopathy in a way that imprinted itself in the minds of all who studied with her. The final section contains the famous 'Brief study Course in Homoeopathy'

HOMEOPATHY IN GENERAL PRACTICE

Dr Alastair Jack, 239pp, 216x138mm, 2001, 0906584515

The practical application of homeopathy described by a general practitioner who has used it extensively for forty years within the National Health Service. Amplified by a critical discussion of 129 cases.

HOMOEOPATHY IN PRACTICE

Dr Douglas Borland (ed. Dr Kathleen Priestman), 208pp, 216x138mm, 1982, 090658406X

The first section deals with homoeopathy in clinical conditions. The second section, 'Studies and Comparisons of Remedies', shows to what extent Dr Borland excelled in leading from one remedy to another, often linking them by their differences or similarities.

HOMOEOPATHY FOR SPORTS, EXERCISE AND DANCE

Emlyn Thomas, RSHom, DPhysED, 337pp, 216x138mm, 2000, 0906584485

Injury and illness are among the most difficult events in the life of athletes, games players and indeed anyone who enjoys physical activity. This book is a reference work for all people who wish to use homoeopathy to help speed recovery.

IN SEARCH OF THE LATER HAHNEMANN

Rima Handley, RSHom, 240pp, 216x138mm, 1997, 0906584353

This is the story of Samuel Hahnemann's practice of homoeopathy in Paris during the last years of his life. It draws on his actual casebooks, and shows him putting into practice the implications of his thinking on chronic disease and experimenting with new remedies. We witness the process of the learning and making of homoeopathy.

INSIGHTS INTO HOMOEOPATHY

Dr Frank Bodman (ed. Dr Anita Davies & Dr Robin Pinsent), 119pp, 216x138mm, 1990, 0906584280

Detailed clinical studies over a wide range of conditions and remedies, including the use of homoeopathy in psychiatry. The author demonstrates that it is possible to subject homoeopathy to the same standards of scrutiny that apply to another branch of medicine.

INTRODUCTION TO HOMOEOPATHIC MEDICINE, 2nd Edition

Dr Hamish Boyd, 285pp, 216x138mm, 1989, 0906584213

A systematic introduction to the principles of homoeopathic medicine. It shows how the homeopath's selection of a remedy is based on a process that is based on the perception of the patient as a whole and individual person.

MATERIA MEDICA OF NEW HOMOEOPATHIC REMEDIES

Dr O.A.Julian, 637pp, 216x138mm, paperback edition 1984, 0906584116

Over a hundred new homoeopathic remedies, for use in conjunction with the classic materia medicas. Some of the remedies are completely new. Others are familiar substances used homoeopathically for the first time.

MENTAL SYMPTOMS IN HOMOEOPATHY

Dr Luis Detinis, 222pp, 216x138mm, 1994, 0906584345

One hundred and ninety-four rubrics relating to rubrics of mental symptoms are studied, drawn primarily from Kent's Repertory, but also from Barthel and Klunker's Synthetic Repertory. Followed by six full case studies.

STUDIES OF HOMOEOPATHIC REMEDIES

Dr Douglas Gibson (ed. Dr Marianne Harling & Dr Brian Kaplan), 538pp, 216x138mm, 1987, 0906584175

These studies differ from any previously published materia medica in their uniquely wide range of insights, combining the panorama of each remedy with a faithful description of the mental and physical symptoms it elicits from a sensitive prover.

TUTORIALS ON HOMOEOPATHY

Dr Donald Foubister, 200pp, 216x138mm, 1989, 0906584256

Offers an insight into Dr Foubister's clinical experience and reflects many of his particular strengths. Detailed clinical pictures, including the use of homoeopathy in paediatrics, with studies on Carcinosin and other remedies.

TYPOLOGY IN HOMOEOPATHY

Dr Léon Vannier, 176pp, 246x189mm, 1992, 0906584302

A study of human types, based on the gods of Antiquity. Discusses the remedies to which the individual types respond best. Fully illustrated with depictions of these types, drawn from classical as well as modern art and sculpture.